Disease Prevention
A Critical Toolkit

John Frank, Ruth Jepson
and Andrew James Williams

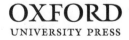

OXFORD
UNIVERSITY PRESS

OXFORD

UNIVERSITY PRESS

Great Clarendon Street, Oxford, OX2 6DP,
United Kingdom

Oxford University Press is a department of the University of Oxford.
It furthers the University's objective of excellence in research, scholarship,
and education by publishing worldwide. Oxford is a registered trade mark of
Oxford University Press in the UK and in certain other countries

Published in the United States of America by Oxford University Press
198 Madison Avenue, New York, NY 10016, United States of America

British Library Cataloguing in Publication Data
Data available

Library of Congress Control Number: 2016932197

ISBN 978-0-19-872586-2

Printed and bound by
CPI Group (UK) Ltd, Croydon, CR0 4YY

To Linda

*from
john*

*(with best
wishes)*

*August,
2019.*

Disease Prevention
A Critical Toolkit

This book is dedicated to the many front line health and community workers the authors have been lucky to have as colleagues, over their careers, as well as our many academic and policy colleagues working to improve public health and reduce health inequalities, around the world. The authors hope this book will provide you with helpful tools to analyse the relative benefits, risks, and costs of preventive interventions proposed in the settings where you live, work, and practice.

Foreword

Whether in clinical practice or in public health, professionals are increasingly being expected to advise the public on claims made for the effectiveness of new preventive medical and community-health interventions. Yet most health professionals are not provided with much training on how to assess the validity of such claims—and particularly on how to critically appraise available scientific evidence on the benefits, risks, and costs of prevention. How can the graduate deal with the daily media diet of bold claims made for preventive clinical manoeuvres, community programmes, and public policies?

This book aims to fill that gap, by providing a basic toolkit to equip the reader for such critical appraisal. Although some of the skills taught in this book overlap with critical appraisal skills of the standard clinical epidemiological sort, the tools of the latter trade often relate purely to the management of ill patients, e.g. critical appraisal of the validity of diagnostic tests, prognostic algorithms, and the (cost-)effectiveness of treatments. By contrast, this innovative book focuses on tools for application to evidence on the prevention of future ill health. The book usefully fills a crucial gap in medical, nursing, and public health specialist education.

Packed full of engaging and informative case studies, the book first takes the reader through the annals of recent medical history, citing occasions when preventive measures were widely adopted prematurely, without adequate critical appraisal—sometimes with major adverse effects at the population level. The authors then proceed to provide, as an antidote to this disturbingly frequent phenomenon, several critical appraisal checklists of questions, supported by clear examples, to enable the reader to analyse the benefits, risks, and costs of any preventive intervention under consideration. They first tackle the foundational issue of appraising of evidence claiming to establish the causation of health outcomes, especially as applied to environmental exposures requiring public health measures for their control (a topic rarely covered adequately in clinical training). The subsequent chapters sequentially cover how to find and assess the quality of structured reviews of prevention's effectiveness, population versus individual level approaches to disease prevention (using the example of obesity), potential pitfalls in the science behind nutritional advice to 'stay healthy', risk factor modification to prevent chronic disease (using statins as a case study), cancer screening (through the worked example of PSA testing for early prostate cancer), and genetic testing to predict future disease risk. The final chapter discusses the crucial issue 'What kinds of prevention are most likely to reduce, as opposed to increase, health inequalities by socioeconomic status?'

Health professionals, as well as the inquiring lay public, will therefore find this volume a useful guide to understanding and more confidently navigating through the dense jungle of prevention controversies, a jungle which is unlikely to disappear anytime soon.

Simon Capewell MD, DSc
Professor of Clinical Epidemiology
University of Liverpool, UK

Preface

The authors have come to believe that preventive medical interventions—and even non-medicalized community public health programmes that implicitly promise health benefits in the future, from actions taken now—all carry a strong ethical requirement of the health professional. He/she must have fully informed themselves of the risks, costs, and benefits of the preventive action, understood them in detail, and then communicated them clearly to individual patients, or entire communities, as appropriate. Otherwise, he/she is guilty of breaking a cardinal rule dating back to the time of the Hippocratic oath: *primum non nocere* ('first, do no harm'). Virtually all health professionals *want* to practice this way, but many simply do not have the knowledge and skills to do so. This is especially true nowadays, when newly-developed preventive advice or interventions are being promoted by scientifically ill-informed special interest groups (of which the authors will give several examples in this book.)

To help remedy this situation, the authors have written this slim volume, which culminates in a tool we have developed to help those about to recommend a preventive action. Recognizing that prevention is an art, as well as a science, the authors hope to support sound decision making, rather than produce hard and fast answers. Throughout the book the authors have illustrated methods for assessing the risks and benefits (and in some cases the costs) of prevention, in many settings. To do this, the authors have included specific examples and 'case studies' to help the reader quickly grasp subtle aspects of evaluating claims for the effectiveness (and sometimes the cost-effectiveness) of a wide range of preventive interventions. Our approach is based on over 40 collective years of teaching research methods to hundreds of graduate students in public health and practising health professionals in related fields, and over five decades of accumulated professional practice. We hope this book is helpful to you, whether you are a clinician, public health worker, or inquiring member of the 'lay' public wishing to know how to critically evaluate preventive tests, procedures, lifestyle advice, and community programmes. We wish you well in that important work.

Acknowledgements

The authors are most grateful to Michelle Estrade MPH, who was kind enough to 'fact-check' and provide detailed edits on Chapters 1 and 5, based on her nutritional science expertise. We also want to thank our families for supporting us during the long process of writing this book, and our funders at the Scottish Collaboration for Public Health Research and Policy, the Medical Research Council of the UK, and the Scottish Chief Scientist Office. Any errors or omissions are, of course, the responsibility of the authors.

Last, but not least, the senior author (JF) gratefully acknowledges the brilliant contributions—over the last three-and-a-half decades—to the art and science of 'critical appraisal' as invented by the McMaster University Department of Clinical Epidemiology and Biostatistics ('CE&B'), in Hamilton, Ontario, Canada, where he was lucky enough to hold his first academic appointment, in 1982–3. Under the initial leadership of the late David Sackett, and then Peter Tugwell (the next Chair of the Department), CE&B developed and perfected what were at that time very novel teaching materials for critically appraising all the main epidemiological study designs used to study the aetiology of disease, as well as diagnostic test utility, prognostication, treatment, and health economic evaluation—focused on *medical care* processes involving patients. The present book owes much to that approach, but focuses entirely on prevention, with consequently much more emphasis on applications of critical appraisal in public health, including interventions directed at entire well populations—as opposed to clinical epidemiology to improve patients' outcomes once they are unwell.

Contents

About the authors

John Frank is a physician/epidemiologist, and Professor of Public Health/ Primary Care since 1982, at four universities in Canada, the USA, and the UK. He has been Professor (now Emeritus) at the University of Toronto, at the Dalla Lana School of Public Health (since 1983), founding Director of Research at the Institute for Work & Health in Toronto (1991–1997), and inaugural Scientific Director of the Canadian Institutes of Health Research—Institute of Population and Public Health (2000–2008). He currently holds a Chair in Public Health Research and Policy at the University of Edinburgh, and directs the Scottish Collaboration for Public Health Research and Policy (www.scphrp.ac.uk). The Collaboration seeks to develop and robustly test novel public health policies and programmes to equitably improve health status in Scotland, through the convening and ongoing support of researcher/research-user consortia.

Ruth Jepson is Deputy Director, Scottish Collaboration for Public Health Research and Policy, University of Edinburgh. After her MSc, Ruth spent over 10 years in the Cochrane Collaboration as a Review Group Co-ordinator and reviewer. She also worked at the NHS Centre for Reviews and Dissemination in York University. She returned to the University of Edinburgh to complete a PhD on developing a measure of informed choice in cancer screening. Prior to 2012, she was co-director of the Centre for Population and Public Health, and lead for the Physical Activity and Diet Research Programme, University of Stirling. Her methodological expertise is in systematic reviews and evaluation research (both qualitative and quantitative), applied to promoting physical activity, through partnerships with service providers and users.

Andrew James Williams is a public health statistician/epidemiologist. He is currently the research fellow in natural experimental approaches for the Farr Institute @ Scotland (http://www.farrinstitute.org/centre/Scotland/ 3_About.html), Scottish Collaboration for Public Health Research and Policy, University of Edinburgh. Originally, he began training in medicine, but transferred out through health informatics into public health. He has a MPH from the University of Birmingham and a PhD from the Peninsula College of Medicine and Dentistry. His research interests relate to the use of non-consented routinely collected data, and child health and wellbeing.

Chapter 1

Introduction: Why we wrote this book

Background

Humans now live for a long time. The Office for National Statistics (2013) predicts that around one-third of the babies born in the United Kingdom in 2013 will live to 100 years of age. This increased longevity is due to a number of advances, including those related to public health successes of the last 150 years (e.g. clean water and sanitation), improved living conditions (e.g. nutrition), reduced family size and increased spacing of pregnancies in time (Ostry and Frank 2010), and the treatment and prevention of communicable disease (e.g. via antibiotics and vaccines).

Consequently, twenty-first century illness and death—in all but the poorest parts of the world—are likely to be due to non-communicable diseases, the causes of which tend to be much more complex, acting over decades. The causes of some of non-communicable diseases span our entire life course, from our inherited genetics and intrauterine exposures, through to the foods we eat and the way we live our lives, encompassing the whole of the social determinants of health (Dahlgren and Whitehead 2007). As a result, to prevent the onset of non-communicable diseases as we age, we need an accurate understanding of the panoply of factors that influence the entire natural history of these diseases, from womb to tomb. Furthermore, we need to understand the detailed process of disease causation, spanning the silent, 'pre-clinical' stages, which are common to most cancers, cardiovascular disease, Type 2 diabetes, and the dementias (to name only the commonest examples), as well as the later stages, during which actual symptoms develop.

The science through which we come to understand these issues, *epidemiology*, uses carefully designed 'cohort' studies of thousands of persons, examined in detail when they are recruited to the study in good health, then followed over many years, until major diseases (or death from them) occur. Statistical analyses are then used to sort out which factors present before disease onset or death, predict those outcomes—so-called 'risk factors'.

Similarly, evaluating whether a specific preventive measure is effective—whether it be in the form of lifestyle changes, vaccines, nutritional supplements or drugs, or even simply having a screening test to detect silent cancers or blood-vessel disease—requires long-term, controlled intervention studies. These studies typically involve tens of thousands of persons followed for many years, ideally randomized (although this is not always feasible, as the authors will show) as to whether they receive intervention or not. Only in this way can science reliably determine whether or not claims made for the effectiveness of specific preventive interventions are valid. Without such evidence, claims made for new sorts of prevention should be considered particularly suspect, simply because they require such an onerous standard of proof.

A conceptual framework for making decisions about prevention

Alongside the evidence from such studies, there are two further perspectives, which need to be considered when deciding upon a preventive action (Fig. 1.1). These will be familiar to those trained in evidence-based medicine.

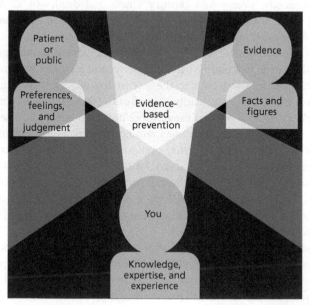

Fig. 1.1 The three perspectives that must come together for evidence-based prevention.

They are the preferences, feelings, and judgements of the individual or community for whom the preventive action is being considered, and your own knowledge, experience, and expertise, as either the health professional involved, or the thoughtful patient or community member seeking an informed decision about proceeding with prevention. Bringing the three perspectives together is much more of an art than a science. Hence, this book aims to provide useful tools and examples to anyone who needs to make a decision about a preventive action, either for professional or personal reasons. Throughout the book the authors have used case studies, particularly recent controversies around 'prevention gone wrong', to illustrate the role of the three perspectives in evidence-based prevention and the sorts of tools that can help bring them together.

Outline of the book

The next chapters use historical case studies to illustrate some of the basic principles of prevention, such as 'the hierarchy of preventive interventions' and the epidemiological methods for assessing evidence of disease causation in human health. These two historical case studies share a number of common features, even though they relate to a non-communicable and communicable disease, respectively pellagra and cholera. Both diseases were of completely unknown causation at the time. The prevailing medical opinion, which ironically favoured an environmental cause for cholera and an infectious one for pellagra, was causing more harm than good, by advocating ineffective control measures. It was pioneering epidemiologists, Joseph Goldberger (1874–1929) for pellagra, and John Snow (1813–1858) for cholera, who were able to use their own knowledge, expertise, and experience, and systematically gathered evidence and identified the correct preventive actions.

Chapter 4 provides guidance on current best practices for finding and evaluating top-quality scientific evidence about disease prevention in the burgeoning global scientific literature, including the assessment of the quality of systematic reviews of the evidence. Systematic reviews, when well done, are a very useful way to reduce the considerable work of finding the best evidence on any effectiveness question, whether of treatments or prevention. The importance of systematically gathering and appraising evidence is illustrated using the example of the commonly held belief that drinking cranberry juice prevents urinary tract infections.

Chapters 5–9 critically analyse a series of modern preventive actions to demonstrate how the failure to integrate the three complementary perspectives of evidence-based prevention (Fig. 1.1) can lead to 'prevention gone wrong'—or, at the very least, divisive public controversy about preventive policies. These case studies also illustrate in detail the hierarchy of primordial, primary, secondary, and tertiary preventive interventions introduced in Chapter 2.

The book concludes, in Chapter 10, by considering one of the most pressing public health concerns of the twenty-first century—health inequality. The authors have reviewed current recommendations regarding prevention to reduce inequalities, which demonstrate that preventive action that seeks to be 'far upstream', usually must be broadly aimed at populations, as well as individuals within those populations, returning prevention to the types of actions Snow and Goldberger used.

The ethics of prevention: 'winners' and 'losers'

Threaded through all the sections of the book, is the fundamental principle that there will be clear 'winners' resulting from most prevention programmes, whose future life is extended, or whose quality of life is improved. There will also be 'losers', who suffer side-effects or personal adverse consequences from being diagnosed with early-stage disease, or with 'being at elevated risk' and perhaps treated for it, but who cannot benefit from that intervention. That lack of benefit can occur for a number of reasons. The first group of 'victims of misguided prevention' do not benefit because they were not in fact destined, in the first place, to ever go on to have the full-blown symptomatic disease before death (because disease prediction is never perfect). Others identified as at risk of future symptomatic disease do not benefit because, undergoing the treatments involves no additional benefits, and carries more risks, than just waiting for the disease to develop and then treating it.

This fundamental uncertainty (reflecting a kind of real-life lottery, but with 'bad-luck tickets' that only yield booby prizes, as well as winning tickets), affects virtually all forms of prevention, including nutritional and lifestyle advice, immunization, and long-term drug therapies for chronic disease risk factors, such as elevated cholesterol or blood-sugar levels, or mild hypertension (which typically cause no symptoms for decades, until complications such as stroke or heart attack develop). Furthermore, more tests and imaging studies are being developed each year, which can detect the pre-clinical disease stages—or even just 'elevated risk'—but, for many of these new detection modalities for very early disease, we do not yet know whether patients will actually be better off as a result of that detection. It turns out that virtually all detection of elevated disease risk, as well as of pre-clinical disease stages, carries risks of its own, as well as significant new costs, as the authors show in Chapters 7 and 8. Together, these phenomena mean that there is an ethical obligation of frontline health professionals and intelligent lay advocates of sound health policy in the modern era, when a proposed preventive intervention requires any significant change in health-related human behaviour. They need to be capable of fully and accurately informing patients—or, indeed, entire communities—about the risks and costs, as well as the benefits of proposed preventive actions. That is why the authors wrote this book.

Chapter 2

Basic principles of successful and unsuccessful prevention

The hierarchy of approaches to effective prevention: the legacy of Joseph Goldberger

In the early decades of the twentieth century, throughout the US 'Old South' and mid-west, a very large, tragic disease outbreak occurred, involving some three million preventable cases and probably more than 100,000 deaths, over three-and-a-half decades. The story of that outbreak—although little known by the present generation of health professionals—has been used by generations of public health instructors and students to teach the basic epidemiological approach to understanding the causes of disease, and then moving on to control the disease, by designing carefully evaluated trials of specific preventive and treatment interventions.

Most people reading this will immediately think of infections as the most likely condition to behave in such an epidemic pattern. In fact, in the massive US outbreak of the early 1900s, it was the strongly held view of the medical and scientific establishment, as well as societal leaders of the time, that the outbreak was infectious in nature. It was the work of one remarkable man, Dr Joseph Goldberger of the US Public Health Service, which proved through a series of creative and brilliant epidemiological studies that the condition in question—pellagra—was not an infection, but rather a nutritional deficiency. Pellagra is caused by a lack of B vitamins in the diet, especially B3 (i.e. nicotinic acid, also known as niacin.) It develops, over months to years, in persons not eating a varied diet that includes naturally occurring sources of the vitamin, such as fresh meat and milk, legumes, and certain green vegetables. And it is particularly associated with diets predominantly consisting of corn. The initial stages are mild, with skin lesions followed by chronic diarrhoea; however, untreated it progresses to irreversible dementia, so that many sufferers ended up in 'asylums for the insane' (to use the language of that time).

This story is retold here because it is still salient for understanding how multi-layered the causes of disease can be, and because it reveals how social context, local culture, and vested interests can readily lead even experts down the wrong path, in identifying the cause of a disease, and therefore in pursuing its successful remediation and prevention. Crucially for this book, the story of pellagra also helps us understand a key principle in epidemiology: multiple points exist at which one can intervene to prevent disease. These range from far 'upstream' interventions, before even asymptomatic disease is present, and thus aimed at the entire healthy population, to more 'downstream' approaches, targeting only persons with full-blown disease, focusing on simply treating them, as new cases arise.

It was 1914 when the US Surgeon General Rupert Blue asked Goldberger to formally take over the investigation and control of the pellagra epidemic, which by that time had affected hundreds of thousands of victims in several states, since its inception in 1906. Goldberger came to the south (he was a Northerner and an immigrant) at a time when a popular local doctor with strong connections to the Old South establishment, Dr James Babcock (previously Superintendent of the South Carolina Hospital for the Insane) had just that year been forced to resign. The accusation against him was that he 'brought disrepute on South Carolina', by exposing to the media, and thus the rest of the USA, the presence and extent of the pellagra epidemic. Initially the outbreak had been covered up relatively easily, since it was first noticed in closed institutions for the mentally ill, prisoners, and orphans. Babcock, who was not a trained public health researcher, had never claimed the disease was anything other than infectious (the dominant view at the time). However, laboratory investigations by highly trained microbiological researcher Dr Claude Lavinter failed to disclose any of the usual characteristics of infectious disease. For example, the condition could not be transmitted in the laboratory to any experimental animal, nor even to human volunteers, for example, by injecting or ingesting samples of tissues and excreta from human cases.

Goldberger began his investigation by touring the worst-affected institutions and neighbourhoods—typically cotton-mill towns where the workers had to buy all their supplies, including groceries, from the 'company store', since only there were they able to buy on credit until their wage packet arrived each month. Within days of his arrival, Goldberger was struck by two facts:

- Even in the worst-affected institutions, there were no cases of the disease among employed staff.
- The main dietary staple in all affected communities was corn meal, biscuits, and molasses, sometimes served with meat, but usually only fatty portions of salt pork.

By the time he reached the end of his initial investigational tour, Goldberger was convinced that the disease was nutritional, and set out to conduct several cleverly designed studies, over the next decade, to prove that hypothesis. The full story of those studies is beyond the scope of this book; the authors recommend a short yet fulsome account by the noted Yale physician Alfred Jay Bollet (Bollet 1992).

Within a short time of Goldberger's initial assessment of the epidemic and its cause, powerful vested interests began to throw their considerable weight against what was to them an appalling notion: that such a terrible scourge could be due to malnutrition. Their sense of outrage was fed by the fact that the disease was previously unknown in the South, and that the diet being implicated as its cause had apparently remained unchanged for generations. There was also a special sense of indignity, in that pellagra only affected the very poorest and most disadvantaged communities in the South, as Goldberger vigorously pointed out, implying that life was profoundly unfair in that part of the USA. Fifty years after the abolition of slavery and the Civil War, which had badly damaged Southern culture and the economy, strong feelings against such external criticism remained. Influential local citizens could not accept that the disease was due to in large part to social conditions; it was less threatening to believe it was caused by an infection.

Goldberger was not satisfied with observational studies, which could only illuminate risk factors contributing to the causation of pellagra. He went on to conduct actual experiments in both its treatment and prevention; these remain models to this day of how public health can move directly into experimental, action-oriented research, whenever the science is adequate to justify a trial of a new intervention's effectiveness (Chapter 3). In 1914–15 Goldberger used federal funds to augment the diet of two orphanages and one part of an asylum for the mentally ill, both of which had very high rates of pellagra at the start of the study. When the annual peak of pellagra cases was expected the following spring, no new cases occurred, and all the old cases had cleared. [This was extraordinary: it is very rare in medicine to show 100% effectiveness for an intervention!] Sadly, the funds ran out and the disease returned the following year, affecting 40% of children at the one orphanage. However, Goldberger's point was made.

In the end, vested interests prevented the acceptance of the increasingly compelling body of scientific evidence, that pellagra was entirely preventable through improving diet. In fact, full acceptance of this fact did not occur until the early years of World War II. Eventually the disease became virtually extinct in the USA, through the provision of Vitamin-B-enriched foods, after the chemical identity of Vitamin B3, and a means of synthesising it in the laboratory, were discovered in 1937. Until then, hundreds of thousands of additional pellagra cases and many deaths occurred in the southern USA—arguably unnecessarily.

This twentieth century pellagra case-study in the US South provides a valuable lesson in prevention, by illustrating at least four hierarchical levels of preventive/treatment intervention. To begin with, three broad categories of interventions could have been used to tackle pellagra effectively using improved diets alone, once Goldberger had shown the way, nearly 25 years before the disease finally died out:

- *Disease control option most 'downstream'*: identify full-blown cases by house-to-house and institutional-resident surveys/examinations, and treat them all with enriched diet (the only treatment that worked, until Vitamin B3 was made available as a medicine, in the 1940s): this approach would be the least expensive in the short run, but would do nothing to prevent further emerging cases in the rest of the population, who would continue to consume the same inadequate diet.

- *Disease control option moderately 'upstream'*: focusing on the communities and institutions with the highest rates of pellagra (thus improving efficiency and reducing programme costs), identify individuals in those settings most at risk of pellagra, based on the risk markers Goldberger identified, such as age, gender, poverty, prior history, and usual diet; enrich those persons' diets, so as to prevent the emergence of new cases before they occur. This approach moves beyond treatment to prevention, but will not prevent all new cases, since some inevitably emerge in settings not identified as high-risk. This moderately 'upstream' option also presents a social acceptability and fairness problem, in that some persons who are not yet actually ill will receive enriched diets, but others (not identified as being at risk) will not.

- *Disease control option most 'upstream'*: consider all the poor residents of the states affected by the outbreak to be at some risk of pellagra, and universally supplement their usual diets with milk, meat, legumes, and other natural sources of Vitamin B3. This option would be the most effective intervention, in that it would prevent virtually all new cases in the affected states' populations. However, it is by far the most expensive and logistically demanding approach, especially when one considers that the Great Depression hit America at about the same time that scientific knowledge of the causes of pellagra was peaking.

The three options described briefly are known as *tertiary prevention, secondary prevention,* and *primary prevention,* respectively (Porta 2008). Throughout this book the authors will return more than once to analogous hierarchy of options in modern preventive policy and programming, for a wide range of diseases.

Remarkably, these same basic preventive/treatment interventions apply to a diverse set of adverse health conditions. Furthermore, they tend to have the same sorts of advantages and disadvantages as have been described for pellagra control. However, in many current controversies in prevention, more distinct *risks are* associated with the interventions promoted to prevent disease than were associated with the generally healthy diets used to stop pellagra. This is especially true for preventive treatments involving:

- ◆ Regular (usually daily) prescription-drug ingestion for years or decades, by persons who may have no disease symptoms (Chapter 7).

- ◆ The invasive treatment of asymptomatic, early-stage disease detected by screening well persons—especially cancer (Chapter 8).

Completing this picture is one even more 'upstream' option for preventive intervention, one often referred to as '*primordial prevention*'. This fourth option comes into play in diseases for which there is clear scientific evidence of a much more fundamental driver of causation. The critical question about the US pellagra outbreak from 1906 to 1940 is why it began *then*. Generations of poor Southerners had indeed consumed an apparently identical diet: corn-meal, biscuits, fat-belly salt-pork, and molasses. Scant formal research exists on this important question. Bollet (1992) points to strong circumstantial evidence that the culprit behind the American pellagra epidemic of that era was a particular change in food processing, which occurred in the USA just after 1900: the development of a new corn-milling machine. The Beall degerminator, patented in 1900–1901, was heralded as an improvement over traditional corn milling with grindstones, because it removed all the germ of the corn, thereby increasing transportability and shelf life, because the fatty content of the corn germ (which is known as corn oil) otherwise goes rancid over time. Unfortunately, many of the most nutritious components of corn are in the germ. In short, the US pellagra outbreak was probably precipitated, in a borderline-malnourished population, by a manufacturing 'advance' that resulted in mass-produced and nationally transported food at cheaper cost, but one severely deficient in key nutrients. This explains why, as Goldberger perspicaciously observed, the cotton-mill towns with monopolistic company stores were much more affected by pellagra than nearby rural residents still milling their corn with traditional grindstones (Fig. 2.1).

Postscripts on pellegra

Ironically, a similar epidemic, involving another dietary staple grain, rice, had taken place in the Far East some 25 years earlier. In the 1880s, the advent of rice-milling machines, through European colonization, led to

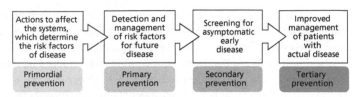

Fig. 2.1 The hierarchy of prevention.

large outbreaks of another Vitamin B dietary-deficiency disease capable of killing its victims: beri-beri. Beri-beri is caused by thiamine (B1) deficiency. Rice milling removes the rice germ, the most nutritious part of the grain, but as with corn it is also the most perishable, because it is the oiliest. Remarkably, one scientist involved in the pellagra outbreak, Casimir Funk, did notice the similarity in the two outbreaks, and published his hypothesis before the conclusion of World War I, but was ignored (Bollet 1992).

As a final post-script, one of the authors (JF) became familiar with pellagra in the late 1970's while working as a Medical Officer in Mbeya Regional Hospital in southwest Tanzania. The disease presented initially precisely as in the Old South: blackened, peeling skin wherever sun exposure occurred. However, it did not proceed as quickly as in Goldberger's time to the more serious manifestations of chronic diarrhoea and finally dementia, presaging death. In the 1970s, we cured all the patients within days, with a simple injection of mixed B vitamins costing only a few pennies. The author (JF) was mindful at the time that we were pursuing mere *tertiary* prevention, and doing nothing to fundamentally change the underlying drivers of the condition's occurrence. Indeed, even our treated patients could expect to present with the same symptoms again in the future, because these water-soluble vitamins cannot be stored in the body long-term. We local physicians passively awaited the annual emergence of new pellagra cases each year, when the village larder was reduced to just corn, before the new harvest was ready, since we were not tackling the underlying nutritional cause of the deficiency.

Years of wider reading about nutrition eventually revealed to the author (JF) the identity of the underlying driver of pellagra in Africa: after Spanish and Portuguese traders brought corn (maize) from the New World in the 1500s, maize-based agriculture gradually forced out more traditional and nutritious staple crops (such as finger millet). Gross caloric yields per cultivated acre were much higher for corn, especially in areas with poor soils and little rainfall. Where is the link here? Why did the adoption of corn as a staple in Africa lead to widespread pellagra, if that was not evident in its New World lands of origin, where native peoples had been eating corn as a staple for millennia? The answer is a testimony to human cultural evolution, and the traditional wisdom of the many indigenous cultures who had survived on corn as their staple for thousands of years, apparently with few ill effects on their health. It turns out that those ethnic groups who traditionally subsisted on corn had a culinary trick, passed down through generations, which renders corn unlikely to cause pellagra if eaten in large quantities, as the staple food in an otherwise limited diet. Nutritional scholars have discovered that the treatment of corn meal with lime (obtained from burning limestone) converts an otherwise un-useable form of the amino acid tryptophan in the corn into a form that can be used by the human body, thus greatly reducing the chance of developing pellagra (Laguna and Carpenter 1951). However, when corn was brought to Africa—by non-agricultural and largely non-cooking slave-traders and other merchants—no one knew to bring along with it the key culinary component of its preparation—lime. Clearly, the effective *primordial preventive intervention* for pellagra in Africa would have been teaching everyone there to cook corn with lime, and/or finding economically feasible ways to diversify the local diet with nutritious locally grown foods, including better sources of B vitamins, such as peanuts and beans.

The moral of the story here is that disease causation is often complex, involving many steps in the causal chain of events. This is especially the case for chronic conditions that come on slowly; and it is these conditions that now cause the majority of premature adult deaths in the developed world, and are rapidly becoming just as important a threat to public health in the poor world (Reddy and Yusuf 1998). When disease causation is complex, prevention can often be tackled in more than one way—some more 'upstream' and bold, but each carrying its own risks and costs.

Another reason to be sceptical of prevention claims: when science gets it wrong

Science finally 'did get it right,' in terms of the cause and control of pellagra, but there have been a surprising number of preventive interventions promoted for wide use in recent decades, which turned out, in the end, to do more harm than good. The scientific errors entailed in promoting and adopting these preventive interventions were not, by and large, *deliberate*. Rather they arose from a combination of two interacting factors.

There is an inherent scientific uncertainty that affects the assessment of prevention effectiveness, especially for conditions occurring well into the future, long after the preventive intervention is initiated. To properly evaluate the effectiveness of such interventions, a *prevention trial* must be conducted, typically by mixed teams of researchers that include epidemiologists and statisticians. In such trials, many persons are formally enrolled, after giving their informed consent to participate, and then followed carefully for some years. There should be two groups of these study subjects, ideally created by randomization (leading to the term 'randomized controlled trial (RCT) more on this later in Chapter 5). One group receives the intervention; a suitable comparison group of similar persons does not receive the intervention (the control group). Then, when a statistically sufficient number of adverse health events, the target of the preventive manoeuvre, have occurred in each group to be sure the results are not due to the play of chance, the rate (i.e. risk) of that adverse health event is calculated in each group, providing direct, empirical evidence as to whether or not the intervention actually reduced the likelihood of developing the disease in question.

There is a natural human tendency, sometimes abetted by vested interests, to jump the gun and *use promising preventive measures prematurely—*before the results of such preventive trials are in. Ideally, these results should be seen to be consistent across independent trials, conducted by different investigators in various settings (as a check against a chance finding due to local circumstances, or unforeseen errors in trial design or analysis.) Unfortunately, such prevention trials often involve closely observing the two groups of subjects (sometimes many tens of thousands of them—more about that later) for many years—due to the low rate of occurrence of the adverse health outcome targeted. Thus there have been several situations where over-enthusiastic physicians, and sometimes even scholarly societies of health experts, have promoted the wide use of a preventive intervention, long before the results of such trials were available, simply because they were so sure, on other scientific grounds, that the intervention 'must work', and therefore 'no eligible patient should be denied it.' In these situations, the eventual completion of controlled trials, or the discovery of previously unsuspected side-effects of the preventive intervention, subsequently demonstrated that many persons were actually harmed, in some cases, more than were helped, by the intervention.[1]

We now turn to four examples of 'prevention science gone wrong', that reveal that even apparently airtight biological arguments for the effectiveness of a disease prevention manoeuvre are no substitute for a properly conducted preventive trial, the 'proof is in the pudding.' Theoretical or basic laboratory science considerations, taken by themselves, are no guarantee that a preventive intervention works, i.e. does sufficiently more good than harm in some persons subjected to it, to balance out the possible lack of benefit, or even actual harm, experienced by other persons. However, the specific mistake made by the medical and scientific community was rather different in each case.

The reversal of medical opinion on hormone replacement therapy (global, 2002–4)

The case of hormone replacement therapy (HRT) reveals how persuasive, but potentially misleading, basic biological science can be in guiding clinical decisions about long-term administration of a chemical substance in healthy persons, in the hopes of health improvement. Female hormones were prescribed, in various forms, to millions of healthy women, either to reduce hot flushes at the menopause, or more frequently, to help preserve feminine body characteristics which normally tend to fade with aging. Let's be clear here: no well-trained clinician would want to withhold such beneficial treatments if their safety were clearly established, especially if they are only administered for a short period of time, specifically for the relief of disabling or distressing symptoms of menopause, but what was happening in some countries, and especially the USA, was that a culturally-normalized demand for 'youth-preserving' HRT developed during the 1970s through the 1990s. As a result, a large fraction of American women in the post-menopausal age group, and their physicians, came to think of HRT administration as a 'normal, natural' way to preserve their femininity indefinitely—some women demanding it from their doctors, others given it as a matter of course by physicians, often with little discussion of potential risks. Those physicians cannot be held entirely responsible, as individuals, for that practice. They were ill-served by the basic medical training of the time, where they had been taught (as had the author (JF)) that such hormones must also surely protect women from the main cause of premature death in women at that time, coronary heart disease. This view was shored up by the well-known delay, about a decade between the onset of most coronary heart disease in women compared to the much earlier onset in men, as they age; it was assumed that female hormones, of the type being prescribed as HRT, were the key cardio-protective factor. However, when the definitive results of the Women's Health Initiative, a pair of huge and well-designed randomized, placebo-controlled trials of the two main forms of HRT then in use, finally came out (Anderson et al. 2004; Rossouw et al. 2002), it was apparent that those randomized to receive the oestrogen/progestin form of HRT experienced an *elevated* risk of heart disease and stroke, as well as blood clots, compared to controls. In hindsight, this was probably because orally administered female hormones had more negative effects on the blood clotting system, which is part of the final stage of arterial blockage in heart attacks and clot-related strokes, than positive effects on the atherogenic process (hardening of the arteries). [This is the process which slowly leads, over decades, to the slow development of narrowed arteries, presaging angina, heart attacks, and sudden cardiac death.] As for the 24% increase also observed in breast cancer risk, no one was too surprised, since many breast cancers had long been known to be hormone-sensitive (i.e. female hormones promote the cancer's growth in certain cases.) In short, the basic science was partly right, but partly dead wrong. And only the large and long Women's Health Initiative trial could, and did, settle the issue. That trial of HRT was stopped some years before planned, because enough excess adverse health events had occurred in the oestrogen/progestin-treated group to be reasonably sure they were not due to chance alone. New clinical practice guidelines, advising against prescribing HRT to well women, based on the trial, were then issued by several authoritative organisations internationally (US Preventive Services Task Force, 2002). Within a remarkably short time, millions of women worldwide had their HRT stopped by their physicians (or simply stopped taking it, on their own, after the trial results became widely publicised.) Unfortunately, calculated estimates of the likely number of heart attacks, strokes, blood clots, and breast cancers caused by HRT, during its decades of widespread use, reveal that many thousands of women probably suffered direct harm as a result of taking it.

Rotavirus vaccine withdrawal (USA, 1999)

In the case of the now-withdrawn, first-generation rotavirus vaccine against infantile diarrhoea, which was marketed in the USA in the late 1990s, a completely different fundamental driver of medical error was operating. All well-trained health professionals know that *rare* side-effects of new vaccines, drugs, and even procedures can never be detected, in a statistically reliable way, by the pre-marketing developmental research, a series of controlled trials that is required in order for legal licensing of the product. Such trials are simply too small, in terms of patient numbers enrolled, and of too short a duration, they are intended to simply assess treatment or prevention benefit, not rare or delayed risks. To clarify, this inherent weakness in our licensing system for new medical interventions occurs for two basic epidemiological reasons.

Rare side-effects cannot be statistically detected with any certainty (the technical term is 'statistical power') with the relatively small trials used to show effectiveness before licensure. If the side-effect is very rare—such as, for example, temporary whole-body paralysis (Guillain-Barre Syndrome), which is known to occur in a few per million recipients of a number of different vaccines—only careful post-marketing surveillance following well-measured health outcomes after use of the vaccine in populations of some millions of people, over some years after its licensure, can reliably detect that side-effect, and estimate its actual frequency. There is no way around this problem. However, most nations could do a better job of setting up post-marketing surveillance systems that would more reliably identify all suspected serious side-effects, such as those likely to cause hospitalization or death.

Side-effects which are long-delayed in their onset, such as cancers or cases of heart disease caused by particular drugs, in a small percentage of those taking them, are particularly hard to identify, even in the most sensitive post-marketing surveillance systems. That is because the lapse of many years between the timing of the side-effect, and exposure to the drug or other product, masks the relationship between the two, too many other events have happened in the interim, also affecting the risk of the adverse health outcome. This tends to muddy the waters, in terms of seeing a clear link between the exposure and the side-effect of a medical intervention. As a result, the sorts of side-effects which are most easily and frequently linked to such exposures are typically rather rare and unusual types of disease, such as rare cancers of particular organs. The rofecoxib story (see Box 2.1 for more detail) is a recent example of a major iatrogenic ('doctor-caused') disease outbreak, from taking a widely used new class of anti-inflammatory drugs (commonly prescribed for osteoarthritis in older people), which only came to light rather late in the game, partly because the diseases caused—or at least accelerated— by the drug, coronary heart disease and/or heart failure, are extremely common in the age-group who were prescribed rofecoxib (trade name Vioxx).

In the case of rotavirus vaccine (RotaShield®), the rare but serious side-effect that came to light after licensure and widespread use was the acute abdominal emergency, intussusception, occurring in approximately one in 5,000 to one in 10,000 healthy infants immunized with this first-generation vaccine. Such a rare side-effect was absolutely impossible to detect with statistical certainty in the pre-marketing trials of the vaccine required by the US FDA, to establish its benefits in preventing diarrhoea. Fortunately, the side-effect is so unusual and dramatic an occurrence in young children, that suspicions were raised very quickly (within months) after the vaccine was released and given to nearly a million infants across the USA, over several months. The Centres for Disease Control in Atlanta, Georgia, quickly mounted case control studies (more about this more complex sort of study of causation is found in Appendix 2) involving hundreds of carefully collected cases of intussusception across the country, and age-matched controls, showing that the former had been much more likely than the latter to have received the new vaccine within the previous few weeks. The agency rapidly recommended against further use of the vaccine, but the manufacturer had already withdrawn it from the market, to avoid both legal suits and damage to their reputation.

Box 2.1 The rofecoxib story: how getting a very common disease from a medical intervention makes it hard to establish causation … and slows regulators' response

In 2004, the international pharmaceutical giant Merck withdrew from the market it's extremely profitable anti-inflammatory drug rofecoxib (*Vioxx*®), after some years of heated arguments between researchers— some convinced of its relative safety and efficacy, and others who pointed to steadily emerging evidence, over the previous half a decade since the drug was licensed for use in the USA, that it caused significant numbers of cases of heart attacks, including sudden cardiac deaths (Karha and Topol 2004). While much has been written about the failure of the drug regulatory system in the USA to promptly act on the scientific evidence of rofecoxib's unintended and serious side-effects, our focus here is on just how faint the 'signal' was that this side-effect actually was real. This is partly because persons likely to take rofecoxib, for garden-variety osteoarthritis related to ageing, are also the sub-population with the highest risk of heart attacks. Because of that risk, the most important studies of rofecoxib's side-effects were large randomized control trials, primarily designed to show that persons taking it suffered less pain, distress, and disability from their arthritis symptoms. Such trials initially only incidentally happened to also measure the rate of heart attacks and sudden deaths, in study subjects randomized to take rofecoxib, compared to those taking an alternative or placebo. These studies culminated in the APPROVe trial, which was actually designed not to assess the impact of rofecoxib on arthritis, but rather the reduction of the development of polyps of the colon, some of which go on to become colorectal cancer (Bresalier et al. 2005). In that study, 2600 patients with prior polyps were randomized to either rofecoxib or placebo, and followed closely for all major illnesses or death for three years. After only half that time, it was noted that the rate of heart attack or stroke among those on rofecoxib was 3.9% versus 1.9% in those on placebo—a doubling of risk, but a difference of only about 26 cases, 1% of the trials' total sample size. The fact that all such outcomes were well counted lent great credibility to this outcome. Furthermore, other sorts of studies found very similar results, when their records were carefully reviewed. In the end, by the time the drug was withdrawn in 2004, it has been estimated by FDA that between 88,000 and 139,000 heart attacks, 30–40% of them fatal, were caused by rofecoxib in the USA alone (Bhattacharya 2005).

As a fascinating account of some of the less-than-scientific factors that played into these decisions, the authors recommend Jason Schwartz' masterful analysis (Schwartz, 2012). That account shows that, while many regard the rotavirus vaccine story as a triumph of science-based public health policy-making, others have questioned the decision-making process that was used to derive the final CDC recommendation to stop using the vaccine. In particular, the decision apparently took no explicit account of the epidemiological estimates at the time of the vaccine's precise health benefits (it was quite effective in preventing serious rotavirus diarrhoea, which is still a cause of many hospitalizations, if only very rarely death, in wealthy countries such as the USA) and risks (composed largely of the much less common side-effect of intussusception). Thus an opportunity was missed to set a precedent for science-based decision-making. Such a precedent, Schwartz argues, could have allowed the vaccine to be ethically marketed to low-income countries even it if it was not suitable for settings with a low risk of death from diarrhoea, such as the USA (although it was in fact priced too high for that, at over USD 100 per infant for all three required vaccine doses). The reason that such marketing would have likely been ethical in these less developed settings, had the price been made affordable, for example: through international development assistance—is that rotavirus diarrhoea kills about 450,000 young children globally (2011 estimate), mostly in sub-Saharan Africa (Tate et al. 2012)—a substantial proportion of all infants born, every year, in poor and remote settings globally. This burden is attributable to a combination of inadequate water supplies and sanitation, and poor access to intravenous rehydration of affected infants, which can usually prevent death if cases are seen early enough. Such large risks of fatal diarrhoeal complications would have made the very small risks of rotavirus vaccine-related intussusception potentially worth taking in these settings, since the vaccine clearly reduced severe diarrhoea by up to 90%.

To step back a bit, a general principle of good medical practice follows from both the rofecoxib and rotavirus vaccine stories: health care professionals and patients should always be wary of *new* drugs, vaccines, tests, and procedures. These are often incompletely evaluated for their risks, until many thousands of patients have used them over several years. Best practice is therefore to reserve the use of new medical interventions for those patients most likely to benefit, in whom potentially unknown risks are likely to be balanced by such benefits. Two such groups of patients commonly qualify, especially those meeting both criteria: those with a particularly high risk of a bad outcome from the condition for which the new intervention is designed; and those who have not responded (i.e. benefited) from the best previously available treatment or investigation for their condition. New preventive interventions for the general population, such as vaccines for very rare or typically mild diseases in the population to be vaccinated, and chronic hormone or drug administration to 'keep people well,' rarely meet these criteria, as these examples testify. Such preventive interventions should always be evaluated by well-designed and executed controlled trials *before* they are recommended for use in, or marketed to, the general population.

Unproven cancer screening: the case of prostate specific antigen testing for prostate cancer

In this third example, a different set of forces combined to drive perhaps the largest single medical error of the century: the wholesale promotion and uptake of unproven screening for prostate cancer, by a high proportion of older men in several developed countries. Widespread use of regular—often annual—prostate specific antigen (PSA) blood-test screening for prostate cancer, in perfectly well older men, began more than two decades before the first rigorous randomized control trial (RCT) could be designed and completed. That trial showed with almost no doubt that this practice causes more harm than good (Schröder et al. 2009). The underlying impetus for such widespread screening, which was far more common in the USA, much earlier than elsewhere, has been a particularly American view of health 'check-ups': that more testing of healthy people is better than less. According to this paradigm, testing can only improve health, since after all, 'any condition detected early will have a better outcome—especially cancer'. As the authors show in detail in Chapter 8, it turns out that this is simply not the case for many diseases, especially some cancers, of which prostate cancer detected by PSA testing is a prime example.

Scared straight (or apprenticeships in crime)

This final example relates to a programme, which wasn't intended to prevent a disease or even a health-related behaviour, but juvenile delinquency. Originating around the early 1970s in the USA, 'Scared Straight' is a well-known example of a type of juvenile delinquency prevention programme, which has been used across the world. Within the programme, youngsters who had already been identified as juvenile delinquents or those considered at risk of juvenile delinquency visit a prison. The purpose of the visit is to expose the youngsters to the reality of crime and its repercussions through interaction with inmates to scare them into 'going straight'. The New Jersey 'Scared Straight' programme was showcased in a television documentary broadcast in 1979. Within the documentary it was reported that success rate was 94% (based on a tiny sample of 17 youngsters) at three months following the visit (Finckenauer 1982). However, when Finckenauer (1982) reported the results of their RCT of the New Jersey programme, not only were participants no less likely to commit crime, they were more likely to be arrested than controls (Petrosino et al. 2013). Further evaluations of similar programmes continued to question their benefits; however, the programme continued to be implemented. Beginning in 2000, systematic reviews of these programmes began to be reported, confirming that the programme increased crime. However, even the 2013 update of the Cochrane review of these programmes continued to find the programme being implemented in some settings. The conclusions of this review read:

> We conclude that programs such as 'Scared Straight' increase delinquency relative to doing nothing at all to similar youths. Given these results, we cannot recommend this program as a crime prevention strategy. Agencies that permit such programs, therefore, must rigorously evaluate them, to ensure that they do not cause more harm than good to the very citizens they pledge to protect (Petrosino et al. 2013, p. 2).

> Reproduced from Anthony Petrosini et al., 'Scared Straight' and other juvenile awareness programs for preventing juvenile delinquency, *Cochrane Database of Systematic Reviews*, Issue 4, Art. No.: CD002796, Copyright © 2013 The Cochrane Collaboration, with permission from John Wiley & Sons, Ltd.

To conclude, there are multiple factors that facilitate errors in science and medicine, when recommending preventive interventions. Some are purely scientific, and largely related to the inherent uncertainty involved in predicting that a given individual will develop a specific health condition, within a particular period of time. Some are more nuanced social, cultural, and economic forces that tend to promote particular views of best preventive practices, but are weak on using hard evidence to back up their case. Others are related to ordinary human nature, with its tendency to be driven by fear of bad outcomes, and to grasp at any straws offered as a means to reduce those risks. Finally, as our last example demonstrates, human behaviour (when that is itself the target of a preventive intervention) is always a challenge to predict, and sometimes interventions to change deviant (or health-related) behaviours can have effects opposite to those intended, leading to more harm than good.

Decision support tool

At the end of the book the authors have presented a generic decision-aid for decisions about prevention, whether it is related to an individual-level clinical manoeuvre, a community programme, or a societal policy (see Appendix 1: Preventive Actions: Decision Support Tool). At the end of this and each subsequent chapter, the authors list which sections in the tool have been discussed, as follows:

Evidence assessment—2B.

Considering the individual, community or population perspectives—2, 3, and 4.

Considering your personal perspective—2 and 3.

Quiz

Suggest an example of an anti-obesity programme/policy for each of the categories of prevention introduced in this chapter, as a hierarchy—primordial, primary, secondary, and tertiary. Which of your exemplary interventions has, in your view, the most potential traction, and which have the least, in terms of the widespread support across society that would be required in order to implement it? [For some suggestions as to answers to this question, have a look at Chapter 5.]

Chapter 3

A brief history of prevention ... and causation

1852, John Snow, and all that—the origins of epidemiology

Epidemiology is often defined as the study of the distribution (in space), dynamics (in time) and determinants of health-related conditions. [At a traditional family picnic, however, the author (JF) has found it easier to just tell relatives that his work involves using statistics to understand 'who gets sick or injured, who gets better and who does not, why, and what can be done about it.']

Epidemiology can be traced back to seventeenth- to nineteenth-century Europeans who first collected data on deaths and populations at risk, in order to calculate rates of death in various settings, and then compare them. Two of these, John Graunt (1620–1674) and William Farr (1807–1883), both in the UK, were among the first population-health scientists, but are more properly considered the first demographers, rather than epidemiologists per se. Their work was, however, ground-breaking in its use of basic statistics about death to infer burdens of disease and premature mortality across the UK, and even across neighbourhoods within one city. These small areas showed marked contrasts in the health and longevity of their residents. For example, Graunt published in 1622, far ahead of his time a systematic analysis (Graunt 1662) of the patterns and rates of death from common, easily diagnosed conditions (e.g. 'excessive drinking', 'grief', and, in infants 'overlaid and starved.') Since routine public sector recording of all deaths was not yet in place (that took until Farr's time, after 1837), Graunt had to organize data collection by older women 'searchers' in each church parish. Using the newly instated universal reporting of vital statistics, Farr compiled routine reports on patterns and trends of UK births and deaths (all expressed as proper rates per thousand persons in the population, per year), showing strong relationships between poverty and premature mortality (Whitehead 2000).[2]

In the middle of the nineteenth century another epidemiological pioneer in Britain was using health statistics to illuminate the causes of a particularly severe epidemic of cholera;[3] he also intervened dramatically in order to stop the spread of new cases. He was the noted English physician and first anaesthetist, John Snow (1813–1858). Snow famously demonstrated that the source of a person's (usually, their household's) drinking water was the main determinant of his or her chances of developing and dying from cholera, which was frequently fatal at that time. John Snow himself comprehensively documented and published his investigations in 'On the mode of communication of Cholera' and there have been numerous subsequent re-analyses.[4] At that time, various private water-supply companies served London. Each company had its main water intake at a slightly different location on the Thames River. Water treatment, such as chlorination, had yet to be invented. Indeed, it was not thought necessary; most medical authorities in the mid-nineteenth century remained unaware of the germ theory of infectious disease. The Vibrio cholera bacteria was not discovered under the microscope until more than three decades later, in 1883, by Robert Koch. In the 1850s, when John Snow was at work, the prevailing belief was that cholera was fundamentally an environmental disease, the result of poor-quality air and soil, especially in damp, low-lying areas, giving rise to disease-causing emanations from the ground called 'miasma(ta).'

Snow calculated rates of cholera deaths occurring in the sets of households served by each water company; he used cholera deaths as his countable outcome, because these were more reliably and completely reported than cases, partly due to the social stigma surrounding cholera. With these data he clearly showed that households nearest a water pump served by the company, with its intake on the Thames just below London, experienced by far the highest rates of cholera death, compared with households served by a water company with its intake upstream of London. Of course, water taken from lower down the Thames was very likely to be contaminated by human sewage, given that no sewage treatment was used at the time. Specifically, Snow found that households exposed to the lower Thames water had 315 cholera deaths per 10,000 households, versus 37 per 10,000 in the unexposed households—an 8.5-fold difference (Morabia 2007; Vinten-Johansen et al. 2003). As we shall see later in this chapter, in our discussion of criteria for establishing causation, this is a very large difference indeed, strongly suggesting, in and of itself, that the causal agent of the epidemic was a contaminated water supply. [Note that there will always be some 'secondary' cases, which have become infected with cholera, not from the water supply, the primary source of contamination, but rather directly from infectious family members and contacts. Thus one cannot expect that 100% of observed cases will be explained by any one source.]

Not limited to statistical methods of data analysis, Snow also collected convincing individual case-studies of persons whose household water supply was almost certainly contaminated by water-borne cholera bacteria, but *who did not become ill*. One group of such protected persons were in fact brewery workers, and therefore unlikely to drink water at all, particularly as they were partly paid in ale and beer. In another renowned case, a woman and her niece died even though they lived some distance from the pump suspected to be contaminated, her sons revealed that she had water from the suspect pump delivered because she preferred the taste (Vinten-Johansen et al. 2003).

Snow's landmark epidemiological investigations were completed in the mid-1850s. However, it was decades before municipal authorities in London and elsewhere acted to systematically improve water quality. When this eventually came about, cholera epidemics were virtually eliminated, as were other largely waterborne diseases, including typhoid fever. Certain medical authorities of the time contributed actively to the delaying of water treatment, delivering public lectures in which they critiqued Snow's theory of cholera causation. The famous German scientist Max Josef von Pettenkofer, used medical meetings as his theatre, where he publicly drank vials of what he claimed were the diluted faeces of cholera patients, and never suffered any apparent harm. We know now that individuals vary greatly in their vulnerability to symptomatic infection by cholera, and indeed many other pathogenic microbes; it is quite possible Pettenkofer was immune, either from prior exposure or innate immunity. It was a convincing challenge to Snow's findings. However,[5] a few years before the major mapping studies of water supply in London were carried out, but after the cholera epidemic had begun, John Snow became famous for an even more prescient act. Using simple maps of cases' homes, Snow reasoned that a particular water pump, at Broad Street (now in Soho), was contaminated. He convinced local authorities to take the handle off the pump, thereby preventing its use. Within days, new cases stopped occurring, as one would predict if one knew what we know now: that the incubation period of cholera (the time elapsed between ingesting contaminated food or water and the onset of symptoms) is a few days in most cases. Snow has thus been dubbed 'the father of epidemiology', not only for his painstaking observational studies to illuminate the cause of cholera, but also for his experimental public health intervention, to promptly act on his observations by shutting down one contaminated water supply at its source.[6]

The key lesson from Snow's work is that he correctly conceived the most important elements of the best observational—as opposed to experimental—study design still universally used by epidemiologists to this day, to identify possible causes of disease or injury: *the cohort study*. Those elements are:

- Establishment of a study population, ideally statistically representative of the real-world population to which the study results are to be applied in public health practice; if individuals are to be individually interviewed and/or examined, they have to provide informed consent to participate in such studies, as in all human-subjects research. Nowadays this must be approved by university or other Ethical ('human subjects') Review Boards before commencing the study.

- Careful measurement of each person's level of exposure to a putative risk-factor—a more general term than 'cause,' as demonstrated below—at the beginning of the study (in Snow's later mapping work, the relevant exposure was measured by the determination of which water company supplied each house, in the neighbourhoods at risk of cholera).

- Assiduous follow-up of all those study subjects—ideally without losing track of any, so as to avoid missing information that may threaten the study's validity—to determine, which subjects develop the disease, injury, or other health outcome of interest.

- Calculation of the rate of occurrence of the health outcome of interest, in the exposed and unexposed subgroups within the study (best done by dividing the count of the outcome events by the total number of person-years of observation in each exposure sub-group, which allows for some persons possibly being followed for longer periods that others).

- Use of statistical methods, as appropriate for the type of outcome examined in the study, to determine whether the observed difference in outcome rates between the two groups is unlikely to be due to chance alone. [Notably, Snow's work preceded the development and widespread use of such statistical testing, but his results showed such a large magnitude (nearly nine-fold) difference between the cholera attack rates in his two large household populations under study, defined by their water supply, that one hardly needs statistics to believe this difference is real.]

Appendix 2, 'Useful resources for a critical appraisal tool kit applied to disease prevention', includes links to the 'critical appraisal tool kits for prevention' that are recommended in this book, in this initial case for assessing the quality of any given *cohort* study claiming to show a causal relationship between a given exposure or risk-factor (whether it is biological, chemical, physical, or even social) and any specific health outcome. It is one of many such 'critical appraisal check-lists' available in both epidemiology texts and on the internet—and one with which the authors have frequently taught, that has stood the test of time.

A further wrinkle: 'association is not causation, but there is a way to tell the difference'

Those of you familiar with controversies in disease causation and prevention will know about the long-fought battle of the tobacco industry to deny that smoking causes lung and other cancers, cardiovascular disease, and more than a half-dozen other diseases for which strong evidence has now accumulated of causation (Glantz 1996). In that long-running debate, a recurring theme emphasized by the defenders of tobacco, is that observational epidemiological evidence of the cohort study sort, *taken by itself*, constitutes evidence only of 'association' not of 'causation' per se. Spokespersons for the tobacco industry are quite correct in that assertion. However, basic training in epidemiology has emphasized exactly this same point for a half-century: showing a strong statistical association between a putative cause and a health outcome in a cohort study (especially only one study) is not in itself sufficient evidence to support an inference of causation. In fact, epidemiologists use a specific 'check-list' to assess whether an *entire body of evidence across scientific disciplines*, about a potential causal relationship in health, credibly establishes causation—a body of evidence that includes, but does not stop at, demonstrating statistical association. As the authors shall show below, using this checklist requires knowing (or finding) and summarizing many sorts of relevant studies, not just epidemiological ones.

Reproduced in Box 3.1 is a recently reworked and updated version of the classic epidemiological 'Criteria for moving from association to causation' (Gee 2008). These criteria were first enunciated by the eminent British occupational and environmental epidemiologist, Sir Austin Bradford Hill (Hill 1965). David Gee, working some forty years later, with the benefit of much more sophisticated epidemiological and environment science in the interim, has cleverly made the original Bradford Hill criteria, since taught to more than two generations of epidemiologists, better suited to assessing evidence of human health effects from *environmental* exposures, including ambient air, water, soil pollution; food contamination; and even physical hazards around us, such as radiation, noise, heat, or cold. Gee's thoughtful and updated version of Hill's original criteria is especially useful in modern times because so many current controversies in disease causation involve such exposures. Environmental exposure can affect very large numbers of people at one time, so that even low individual health risks from such exposures can add up to very large societal burdens of illness, because of the large numbers of persons affected (as shall now be shown).

Box 3.1 The Bradford Hill 'criteria' (Hill 1965) for helping to move from association to causation, with some illustrative examples from the European Environmental Agency report 'Late Lessons from Early Warnings' as cited by Gee (2008).

1. *Strength of the association?* John Snow found 315 cholera deaths per 1000 houses served by polluted water, but only 37 per 10,000 houses served with sewage-free water (London 1854).

2. *Consistent results?* The US Surgeon General Report in 1964 found 36 studies linking smoking with lung cancer.

3. *Specific effects?* In 1959, the then rare cancer, mesothelioma, was observed to kill children in South Africa who played on asbestos waste tips without there being increases in other causes of their death.

4. *Temporality?* 'Is the cart coming before the horse'? The diethylstilbestrol (DES) exposure of mothers occurred before rare cancers in their daughters were observed (USA, 1970).

5. *Biological gradients?* Does the effect increase with dose, if such exposure measurements are available? Lung cancer risks were found to rise steadily with the number of cigarettes smoked per day, in initial studies nearly 65 years ago (UK and USA, 1950s).

6. *Biological plausibility?* Depends on the 'knowledge of the day', and may change over time, as the observation may be new. For example, polychlorinated biphenols (PCB) contamination of eagles (Sweden, 1966).

7. *Coherence?* Is the evidence coherent with the general known factors? For example, radiation damage from X-rays (USA, 1904). Also dependent on the knowledge of the day.

8. *Experiment (reversibility)?* Does prevention prevent? For example, a reduction of SO_2 eventually leads to less lake/forest acidification (Sweden, 1998).

9. *Analogy?* For example, collapsing fish stocks from over-fishing in different areas (e.g. California sardine collapse, 1942, was a useful lesson for other fish stocks).

Adapted from Gee D., 'Establishing evidence for early action: the prevention of reproductive and developmental harm', *Basic & Clinical Pharmacology & Toxicology*, Volume 102, Issue 2, pp. 257–66, Copyright © 2008 Nordic Association for the Publication of BCPT (former Nordic Pharmacological Society), with permission from John Wiley & Sons Ltd. Source: data from Poul Harremoës et al., *Late lessons from early warnings: the precautionary principle 1896–2000*, European Environment Agency, Copenhagen, Denmark, Copyright © EEA 2001.

The following comments provide more detailed advice to the user of the Gee version of the Bradford Hill criteria, to be used as guidelines for assessing claims of causation in human health, especially for environmental exposures:

Strength of association

The first criterion ideally requires a summary estimate—across many studies of the same question (see 'Consistent results' below)—of the *difference* in risks of the health outcomes under study (known as the 'attributable risk' or AR) between persons exposed and persons not exposed to the putative hazard/cause of illness. However, to enable comparisons of the strength of association across different studies, of differing designs in a range of diverse settings, epidemiologists usually calculate the 'relative risk' (RR: one risk *divided by* the other) of the health outcome in question, comparing exposed and unexposed study sub-populations. [The example we have already seen is Snow's calculation of cholera death rates in households with a contaminated water supply, and those without. The attributable risk of cholera from this exposure—during a second outbreak Snow studied was (171 minus 5) = 166 per thousand households; the relative risk was 171/5 = 17.2].[7] The AR (also termed the 'risk difference') tells you how many extra cases of the outcome in question occur, for example, per thousand population, per year, if everyone is exposed to the potential hazard under study. The AR reflects the relative public health importance of the illness caused by the exposure. It does not take into account the frequency of the causative exposure itself in the entire population, for which a slightly more complicated formula is required: the proportion of the health outcome in an entire population, which is attributable to the exposure, termed 'Population Attributable Risk' (Fig. 3.1).

Relative risk, on the other hand, has no units, and reflects purely the 'strength' or 'magnitude' of the association under study, in terms of the causal 'force' linking the exposure and outcome. For example, epidemiologists often quote the classic early studies of lung cancer and smoking (Doll and Hill 1950) as demonstrating a 'strong' association, in that moderate to heavy smokers were found to be at about 3 to 30 times the risk of lung cancer as non-smokers, depending on how many cigarettes they smoked per day, and for how long. On the other hand, most chronic diseases have multiple risk factors, each of which tends to have a rather modest strength of association with the disease, but which combine with effects of other risk factors, in the many persons in modern populations who have more than one, to create quite large relative risks overall for such individuals. For example, smoking, moderately high cholesterol, and moderately high

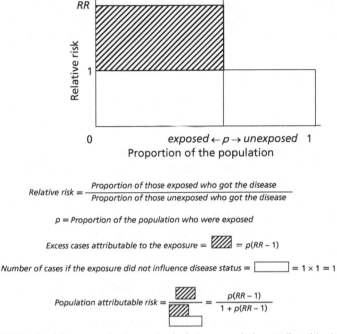

Fig. 3.1 Method for remembering and calculating population attributable risk.

blood pressure each have a relative risk of only 2 to 3 for coronary heart disease (CHD) (National Institute for Health and Care Excellence, 2014). However, a person with all three risk factors has a relative risk of CHD of 6 to 9, depending on his/her precise total risk-factor profile, compared to a person with none of the three. An extreme example, and one of the highest relative risks ever documented by an epidemiologist, is 223, shown by R. Palmer Beasley et al. (1981) for the association between having chronic hepatitis B viral infection and subsequently developing a specific cancer of the liver, hepatocellular carcinoma. This is the equivalent of saying that this disease almost never develops in persons who are not infected with hepatitis B, and is extremely frequent in persons who are thus infected. Such strong 'specificity' (see 'Specific effects', below) of disease causation is common in infections, single-gene diseases (Chapter 9) and some chemical-exposure related diseases. But it is not at all common in the major chronic diseases: the common cancers, diabetes related to being overweight and cardiovascular diseases. Indeed, for the major chronic diseases, we expect risk factors we identify from now on, through new studies, to have relatively low RRs (often less than 1.5), simply because most of the stronger-association risk factors, such as smoking, excess weight, high blood pressure, and elevated cholesterol levels, have already been discovered, and are currently the target of evidence-based programmes in clinical and public health practice to detect and manage them.

Consistent results

This criterion explicitly requires the identification of all the best-quality studies done to date of a given association, in order to extract from each of them the estimate of the RR linking the exposure and outcome in question. Thus, to an even greater extent than is the case for the first criterion, the second criterion cannot be addressed without systematically reviewing the relevant scientific literature, and then using modern methods of statistically combining RR estimates from several studies, a form of *meta-analysis*. This topic warrants its own chapter for a very good reason (Chapter 4). The ability to summarize numerous studies of one question assumes other prerequisite skills:

◆ The ability to first find these studies in the literature.

◆ Being able to then critically appraise their quality (for example using the check-list of questions for cohort studies found in Appendix 1).

◆ The ability to summarize (ideally, statistically) what they say.

To further complicate matters, it is not always appropriate to summarize estimates of the same exposure-outcome RR across studies—for example, when the various pertinent studies use widely varying analytic methods, and/or differing exposure and outcome measures (see Chapter 4 for details).

Specific effects

As implied above in the use of the hepatitis B and hepatocellular carcinoma example, where the RR is 223, occasions arise where a particular exposure is the only known cause of a very specific disease. To take another example, both the serious pulmonary condition asbestosis, and mesothelioma, an aggressive tumour of the lining of the lung and of other body cavities, are almost exclusively caused by exposure to asbestos (Ledingham and Warrell 2000). Epidemiologists generally appreciate that such specificity between exposure and outcome is highly convincing evidence of causation *when it occurs*, but we know that this does not happen often in the commonest human diseases and risky exposures. For example, smoking contributes to the causation of dozens of diverse diseases, but virtually all of them have other causes as well. Thus, this criterion is relatively strong evidence of causation when it is met, but unhelpful when it is not met (i.e. it is a sufficient but not necessary criterion).

Temporality

While seemingly obvious, this criterion has the important role of preventing one from concluding that causation is present when the exposure or risk factor in question develops *after the onset of the disease in question.* For example, chronic mental illness is often associated with socio-economically deprived environments. Yet, the severe mental illness schizophrenia appears to have about the same lifetime probability of occurrence (about 1% of the entire population) in widely varying societies and settings (Sartorius et al. 1986). Health professionals sometimes assume that low socio-economic status, because it has been shown to be a genuine risk factor for so many diseases, is a genuine risk factor for schizophrenia, in the sense that it truly contributes to the disease's causation. However, many studies over decades have established that the actual occurrence rate for this disabling condition is not in general differential by social class. Rather, persons who develop the condition typically experience downward social mobility, often into actual poverty, within a few years of the disease's onset (usually in the late teens or twenties). In fact, often their families experience a downward slide in socio-economic status as well, due to the disease's stigma and the costs of supporting adults disabled by schizophrenia. In short, while schizophrenics and their families often experience deteriorating socio-economic circumstances in the years after the disease develops, its occurrence per se is not strongly related to the socio-economic status of the family before that time (Goldberg and Morrison 1963).

Biological gradients (also called 'dose–response relationship')

This criterion asks whether different levels of exposure to the potential health hazard, or risk factor under study, show different strengths of association, in terms of RR of the outcome in question. For example, in the early studies of lung cancer and smoking, the RR for developing the cancer, compared to the risk in non-smokers, was about 2.5 for light smokers, about 11 for heavy smokers, and nearly 30 for chain-smokers (Wynder and Graham 1950). When it is possible to divide up the exposed subjects in a cohort study (or alternatively, a case control study—see Appendix 2) into those with clearly varying levels of exposure, the finding of such an ordered relationship, between three or more levels of exposure and the RR of the outcome at each level, is generally regarded as strong evidence of causation. However, some sorts of exposure are inherently binary: all or nothing. For example, suppose a rare brain condition in later life is found be more common in outdoor workers and golfers, leading to the hypothesis that being struck by lightning in mid-life is a risk factor for this disease in later life. Even if one could find enough cases of the disease, and a population at suitably high risk of lightning strikes, one would not be able to look for a dose-response relationship, since being struck by lightning is more or less an all or nothing phenomenon. In this sort of 'binary exposure' situation, 'Temporality' simply does not apply.

Biological plausibility

This criterion asks: is there a clear and plausible biological mechanism by which the exposure under study could cause the health outcome? Applying the criterion in practice is more difficult since it depends on:

◆ The extent of the assessor's biological knowledge relevant to the causation question under consideration.

◆ Current scientific knowledge in that area, which is constantly changing.

When expert panels are convened to assess causation, as has occurred for example in the case of second-hand tobacco smoke and breast cancer, the panel typically includes a well-known laboratory-based biologist who is expected to cover off this criterion (Miller et al. 2007). That biological evidence is then made explicit in the resulting structured review of all the evidence in favour of causation (or not) for that exposure and outcome.

Coherence

As with 'Consistent results', applying this one requires an assessment of virtually all high-quality scientific studies to date, relevant to the question: 'Is the putative causal relationship consistent with the overall descriptive epidemiology of the condition, in terms of its times and places of occurrence, and the sub-populations known to be at high risk?' Only an expert in the health outcome under study (e.g. breast cancer), and/or the exposure in question (e.g. second-hand smoke) can properly make this assessment, in light of current scientific knowledge.

Experiment (reversibility)

In many ways this is the most important criterion, from the point of view of practical prevention; it asks 'Is the removal of exposure to the putative causal exposure/risk factor proven to reduce the subsequent risk of developing the outcome in question?' For example, in their landmark study of UK physicians who quit smoking, Doll and Hill (1964a,b) were able to show that those doctors' chances of developing lung cancer, declined rapidly for each year since their last cigarette. This decline in risk was large and relatively rapid, starting from a RR (compared to 'non-smokers') of over 18 in non-quitters; dropping to just under 10 in those who had stopped for less than five years; dropping further to 7 if they had stopped 5–9 years earlier; and plateauing at less than 3 for those who had stopped for more than a decade. It is noteworthy that the benefits of quitting smoking, at least in terms of reducing the risk of lung cancer, are both quite large and rapid enough for even older smokers to benefit from quitting. The risk reduction pattern after quitting smoking is not quite the same for the risks of other health outcomes causally linked to tobacco:, such as chronic obstructive pulmonary disease and CHD, which both tend to show more rapid and complete reversal of risk, although this is not the case once severe lung complications of decades of smoking are present, the damage to the lung is too great. There is some less optimistic news though, about reversing lung cancer risk after quitting; at least within the period of observation covered by the Doll and Hill study, those risks never really seemed to return to the level of life-time non-smokers. This is biologically plausible, since some lung cancers, like many other cancers, appear after *decades* of exposure to the relevant carcinogen. Mesothelioma can occur over 50 years after short-lived asbestos exposure. The truth is, therefore, that some risks are never fully reversible, even after eliminating all hazardous causal exposure; the body sometimes has just too long a memory. However, when some degree of reversibility can be demonstrated, as with the Doll and Hill study, this is valuable additional evidence for causation.

Analogy

This criterion means, 'Is there a comparable condition, perhaps in another animal species, which is also probably caused by the same exposure, and for which we have strong evidence of causation, across the above eight criteria?' When one can find such analogies, they are indeed valuable, but not finding an analogy is not sound evidence against causation, because the biology of each species is to some extent unique, and many human diseases have no precise animal counterpart. An example is scurvy due to vitamin C deficiency: almost all mammals can synthesis vitamin C in their bodies from foods that do not contain it. Evolutionary studies have yet to discern why humans and guinea pigs are among the few exceptions.

The criteria for causation listed above were not intended by their originator, Bradford Hill, to be rigidly applied. Across the nine criteria, there is no recommended minimum number, which must be met, in order for an exposure to be deemed a 'definite' cause of a health outcome. Rather, they are meant as guidelines, to help us make a qualitative judgement on the overall current evidence for and against causation, at any given point in the history of studying any potentially causal relationship in human health. Sometimes that evidence changes so dramatically over time that entire communities of global experts in a field reverse their position on an issue. Environmental (second-hand) tobacco smoke (ETS) was deemed as late as the mid-2000s, by expert panels in more than one setting, *not to* be causally linked to breast cancer (Roddam et al. 2007). However, with the publication of the landmark summary (meta-analysis) of all the previous epidemiological studies on the question, by Miller et al. (2007), opinion began to shift. Now most experts believe that significant exposure to ETS, especially in younger women (and perhaps particularly those who have not yet been pregnant, in whom breast tissue may be more susceptible to inhaled carcinogens) more than doubles a woman's chances of developing breast cancer. This is not a trivial finding. Millions of women worldwide are exposed to second-hand tobacco smoke every day, especially in countries with no legislation prohibiting smoking in workplaces and public venues).

Decision support tool

*Evidence assessment—*2A.

*Considering the individual, community or population perspectives—*3.

*Considering your personal perspective—*2 and 3.

Quiz

In the USA over two decades ago, a new and frequently fatal disease began to strike down women of reproductive age, after only a short illness: 'toxic shock syndrome (TSS)'. Pathology and clinical studies suggested that the culprit was a bacterial toxin absorbed into the body from a mucous membrane, but because the condition was so rare (only some dozens of cases had occurred when the first epidemiological study on causation was done), a cohort study was not appropriate; only a case control study (Appendix 2) could identify potential risk factors for the condition. This study clearly suggested that use of a particular brand of menstrual tampon was the exposure that led to TSS (Todd et al. 1978). In fact, because the study found that *all* the TSS cases had used the implicated brand of tampon, compared to only 26% of the healthy controls, the estimated RR (strength of association) between this exposure and the outcome TSS was effectively infinity. However, the absolute risk of acquiring TSS, related to the use of that brand of tampon, was very small, suggesting that there must have been other key factors operating, besides use of the implicated tampon brand, that combined to cause the disease. What do you think may have been the legal arguments used by the lawyers acting for the manufacturers of this tampon, in defending their clients from civil litigation brought against them by TSS victims and their families? How would you respond?

Chapter 4

Seeing the forest for the trees—finding and using the evidence

Finding the evidence to help make decisions about public health interventions

In the last few decades there has been increasing interest in establishing the effectiveness, and cost-effectiveness, of health care interventions including those relevant to public health. This has resulted in a vast number of evaluation studies, undertaken all over the world (although primarily in North America, Europe and Australasia), and published in one of the 7,000 or so medical or health care related peer-reviewed journals. Still more studies and evaluations (including PhD or Masters level work) may never make it into the peer-reviewed literature; their reports often end up on websites, on office shelves or in local libraries. The latter type of evidence is often referred to as 'grey literature' and can be difficult to find as it is not indexed in electronic databases such as MEDLINE or PubMed.

For the practitioner or lay person, it is daunting to search the Internet or a health database for a topic area, and be confronted with tens of thousands of 'hits', including numerous websites offering evidence summaries and/ or providing guidance. There are, however, several trustworthy organizations that exist specifically to summarize and make sense of all the research, and make judgements for practitioners and decision-makers on, which are effective and of good quality. There are also organizations, which produce evidence-based guidance (see 'Cochrane Database of Systematic Reviews (CDSR)'). Before describing these sources, it is important to provide a brief introduction to 'the best' type of research studies to ascertain the effectiveness of an intervention, programme or service.

Generally, the best way to establish whether an intervention is effective (or not) is to undertake a randomized controlled trial (RCT). A RCT is designed in such a way to minimize bias that can occur, and ensure that any benefits or harms can be attributed to the intervention itself. An important caveat, however, is that RCTs are usually only undertaken where there are areas of uncertainty. When there is clear evidence of beneficial effect (for example, that clean water reduces the incidence of certain types of diarrhoea), RCTs are unethical and unnecessary. However, an RCT is likely to be necessary to determine the most effective way of providing clean water (e.g. filtration or disinfection or a combination).

RCTs are not appropriate for all public health interventions (especially ones, which have many different components, or are implemented at a population level) and so other designs such as natural experiments or 'quasi-experimental' (e.g. before and after) studies are used (John Snow's examination of cholera, considered in Chapter 3, is considered an early natural experiment. These will be discussed in more detail in Chapter 5). RCTs and other 'number' studies (called quantitative studies) are also not very helpful in answering important questions such as 'How does this intervention work', 'Why does it work for some people and not others', and 'What is going on, why isn't my intervention working?' For these sorts of questions, qualitative studies or other types of evaluation can be particularly insightful, coverage of which is beyond the scope and scale of this book (see Patton 1990; Pawson 2013; Pawson and Tilley 1997).

To date, tens of thousands of RCTs have been undertaken, and in the late 1980's it became clear that there was a need to summarize what was known from all the RCTs on a particular topic area, and make these summaries useful to decision makers. For example, if only one RCT showed that filtration was effective for creating clean water, a practitioner might have questioned whether it was likely to work in their specific setting. However, if several studies undertaken in many different settings, had been summarized, and they all showed that filtration was effective, the practitioner would have greater trust in their potency (for a systematic review on this topic area, see Clasen et al. 2006).

The most reliable way of summarizing studies[8] of effectiveness (primarily the RCT) is the systematic review. Systematic reviews are literature reviews that use transparent, reproducible methods, to identify, quality assess, and summarize the findings from studies. Their topic area can range from being very broad (e.g. assessing all interventions to increase the uptake of any health screening) to much more specific (e.g. assessing the effectiveness of leaflets to increase the uptake of cervical screening). The most credible, high-quality and up-to-date source of systematic reviews is The Cochrane Library, which is freely available in many countries (http://www.thecochranelibrary.com/). The Cochrane Library is an on-line, continuously updated collection of six databases that contain different types of high-quality, independent evidence to inform health care decision-making. The most well-known of these databases, and perhaps the most important for people new to systematic reviews, is the CDSR.

Cochrane Database of Systematic Reviews

This database contains thousands of reviews, on many different health care topics (not just public health). Cochrane reviews are often judged to be amongst the highest quality systematic reviews, and should be the first place when looking for evidence for the effectiveness of a particular intervention. They cover the whole of health care from medical and surgical interventions to behavioural and legislative public health interventions. There is a Cochrane Public Health Review Group (Doyle and Cochrane Public Health Group 2009) and CDSR can also be searched by Topic Area or special collections such as Malarial Control to identify relevant reviews. Cochrane reviews have several important features, which ensure their quality and timeliness and are designed specifically to minimize bias being introduced, either by the researcher undertaking the review, or by the evidence included in the review:

1. *They use transparent and reproducible methods to identify, which studies should be included.* They clearly state how they identified studies and how they decided which to include and exclude. This transparency ensures that the researcher does not just include studies, which support or refute their own opinions and beliefs on the topic of interest

2. *They primarily include the highest quality efficacy and effectiveness studies (RCTs).* Up until the last 10 years the focus of Cochrane reviews was only on RCTs. However, other evaluation designs are now included as mentioned previously, RCTs are the design of choice for measure the true effect of any intervention.

3. *Authors must publish a protocol prior to publishing the full review.* All Cochrane reviewers have to first publish a protocol, in which they specify how the review is going to be undertaken. Once this has been peer reviewed and published, the reviewers can then proceed with the review. Publishing a protocol ensures that a reviewer does not go 'off track' when they find evidence, and so should reduce author bias.

4. *They are updated every two years or when new evidence accrues.* Because Cochrane reviews are published electronically, they can be updated whenever new evidence emerges. So, for example, if a new study of the effectiveness of an intervention to increase cervical screening is published, it can be included in the review of that topic. This sort of updating is not possible (at the time of writing this book) in reviews published in other journals or databases.

Box 4.1 Efficacy, effectiveness, and efficiency

These terms are similar but have very different meanings and implications

Efficacy measures how well an intervention works under 'ideal circumstances' (usually in research trials). For example a randomized controlled trial (RCT) can be designed to establish whether an educational intervention can help people to eat more fruit and vegetables. The trial may find that the intervention increases fruit and vegetable intake by two pieces a day.

Effectiveness relates to how well a treatment works in practice. Efficacy of an intervention demonstrated in an RCT does not necessarily translate into effectiveness when implemented in the real world. Often the effects of an intervention are smaller in the real world than they are in clinical trials. So people using the educational intervention in the real world may only increase their intake by 0.5 pieces a day.

Some RCTs do try to measure effectiveness by undertaking the research in a real life setting. However, people are still likely to behave differently when they are in a research situation.

Efficiency measures whether resources are being used to get the best value for money. Using the educational intervention as an example, the question may be asked: Is it more efficient (value for money) to spend money on educational interventions or on increasing the availability of low cost fruit and vegetables?

5. *They are peer reviewed.* As with many other journal articles, they are peer reviewed which means that they have had a least one academic giving critical feedback on the review.

6. *They use specialized software.* They are all published electronically, using specialized software, which means that they are standardized, and use the same terms and expressions in their reporting and analyses.

An emphasis is placed on 'translating the evidence' (which can be hard to understand) into a plain language summary (which are specifically designed for the lay audience). This is a useful place to start for a general overview of the evidence. It provides details of the quality of the RCT evidence, and whether the interventions are effective or ineffective. Figure 4.1 demonstrates how to read a lay summary of a Cochrane review of 'Interventions targeted at women to encourage the uptake of cervical screening' (Everett et al. 2011).

For some readers, this summary may provide them with all the information required. However, a practitioner who wants to deliver an intervention

Describes the topic area that the review covers

- *'Cervical cancer is the second most common cancer world-wide. Increasing the uptake of screening is of great importance in controlling this disease through early detection and treatment of pre-cancerous changes before malignancy evolves'* (p. 87).

Describes the interventions that the review is going to consider

- *'Methods of encouraging women to undergo cervical screening include invitations, reminders, education, message framing, counselling, risk factor assessment, procedures and economic interventions. These were all examined in this review'* (p. 87).

Describes the results of the review

- *'There was sufficient evidence from good quality RCTs to support the use of invitation letters in increasing the uptake of Pap smears. There was also some evidence to suggest that educational interventions may increase Pap smear uptake. Overall, educational materials appeared promising, but it is unclear without evidence from additional good quality RCTs which methods (i.e. printed, video/slide or face to face presentations) are most effective'* (p. 26).

Describes the conclusions of the review

- *'A number of other interventions including revealing the gender of the smear taker and using a health promotion nurse appeared to be promising approaches, but their effectiveness was only examined in a limited number of trials. Likewise interventions by lay health workers appear to be promising in improving uptake, although the number of trials in this area is limited. Overall, these findings relate to screening in developed countries and their relevance to developing countries is unclear'* (p. 26).

Fig. 4.1 How to read a lay summary of a Cochrane review.

Text extracts reproduced from Everett, T. et al. 2011, 'Interventions targeted at women to encourage the uptake of cervical screening', *Cochrane Database of Systematic Reviews* 2011, Issue 5. Art. No.: CD002834, Copyright © 2014 The Cochrane Collaboration, with permission from John Wiley & Sons, Ltd.

may need to read the section at the end of the review called 'Implications for Practice.' In this review of screening for cervical cancer, the authors' state:

> There was sufficient evidence from good quality RCTs to support the use of invitation letters in increasing the uptake of Pap smears. There was also some evidence to suggest that educational interventions may increase Pap smear uptake. Overall, educational materials appeared promising, but it is unclear without evidence from additional good quality RCTs which methods (i.e. printed, video/slide, or face to face presentations) are most effective . . . Overall, these findings relate to screening in developed countries and their relevance to developing countries is unclear.

> Reproduced from Everett, et al. 2011, 'Interventions targeted at women to encourage the uptake of cervical screening', *Cochrane Database of Systematic Reviews* 2011, Issue 5. Art. No.: CD002834, Copyright © 2014 The Cochrane Collaboration with permission from John Wiley & Sons, Ltd.

The implications above suggest that invitation letter can increase uptake of cervical screening and should be used as a first choice intervention. Other interventions may be implemented, but the practitioner needs to be aware that their effectiveness has not been evaluated in enough studies. This does not mean that they are ineffective, but only that there are not enough high-quality studies for the reviewers to be confident about the 'true effect' (see Box 4.2).

There may be some limited evidence of effectiveness available and it is worth looking at the results of the review in more detail to see whether there are any studies that have been undertaken, and whether there may be some benefit (and what the potential harms are, if any). Cochrane reviews, as well as presenting summary results of RCTs, also provide some rich information on the RCTs themselves.

Although there are currently over 8,500 Cochrane reviews, there are still many topic areas that have not been covered. A practitioner interested in social interventions may also wish to search The Campbell Library, which is compiled by the Campbell Collaboration. The Campbell Collaboration is an international research network that produces systematic reviews of the effects of social interventions and uses similar methods to the Cochrane Collaboration, but undertakes systematic reviews in education, crime and justice, social welfare, and international development. Some of these topics are relevant to public health, as they may be interventions which impact on health.

If there is not a Cochrane review in the relevant topic area, there are several other databases that can be searched such as the Database of Reviews of Effectiveness (Centre for Reviews and Dissemination 2015) and Health Evidence.

Box 4.2 Evidence of no effect vs. no evidence of effect

A very important concept to understand is the difference between evidence of no effect and no evidence of effect. These are two very different statements which are often confused.

'Evidence of no effect'

Means that enough high-quality studies have been found and their combined results show that the intervention is no more effective than the control. So, for example, a structured review may find that there is conclusive evidence that an intervention was no more effective than doing nothing—this implies that there was enough sample-size/statistical 'power,' across the studies summarized, to rule out an effect large enough to be of public health interest.

'No evidence of effect'

Generally means that no studies (or only a few studies) were found and the reviewers were not able to say whether the intervention was effective or not. This is a relatively common finding, and may apply to new interventions, where no studies have been done. This statement, therefore does NOT mean that the intervention is ineffective, just that we don't know yet (the jury is out). In these circumstances, it is common for the reviews to state that, 'more research is needed' which can be frustrating for a practitioner who wants to know how to proceed now, not in a number of years.

Database of Abstracts of Reviews of Effectiveness

DARE is focused primarily on systematic reviews that evaluate the effects of health care interventions and the delivery and organization of health services (Centre for Reviews and Dissemination 2015). The database also includes reviews of the wider determinants of health such as housing, transport, and social care where these impact directly on health, or have the potential to impact on health. It is produced by the University of York, UK, and is available free of charge. These abstracts (of systematic reviews) are written and independently checked by researchers with in-depth knowledge and experience of systematic review methods. Each abstract contains a 'bottom line' summary of the topic, findings and reliability of the conclusions. Brief details are then given of the review methods, the results, conclusions and, uniquely a critical assessment of the methods used and the reliability of the conclusions drawn. The purpose of this commentary is to help users of the database to judge the overall validity and reliability of the review.

Health Evidence™

Health Evidence™ is a Canadian database that is similar to DARE in that it also performs quality assessment of systematic reviews, but its focus is primarily public health interventions (McMaster University 2015). At the time of writing the database contained over 4,000 quality-rated systematic reviews evaluating the effectiveness of public health interventions. The producers of the database search the published literature and compile public health relevant reviews, eliminating the practitioner's need to search and screen individual databases.

Reviews of qualitative evidence

In recent years, there has been increasing recognition that insights from qualitative studies can provide a greater understanding on a range of questions, which are not about the effectiveness of the interventions. Typical questions may ask the following:

What? E.g. what are the views of people towards fluoridation?

Why? E.g. why do some women breastfeed, whilst others do not?

How? E.g. how do people respond to an advert on healthy eating?

The Cochrane Library is starting to publish reviews of qualitative studies, but the numbers are relatively small. To find reviews of health promotion studies, a good source is the EPPI-Centre[9] (Social Science Research Unit 2009), which has been at the forefront of this work for many years. The EPPI-Centre conducts systematic reviews in four major areas:

- ◆ Education and social policy.
- ◆ Health promotion and public health.
- ◆ International health systems and development.
- ◆ Participative research and policy.

Although the previous sections have suggested that it is relatively easy to find summaries of the effectiveness of preventative interventions, occasions arise when there is conflicting evidence from these summaries in the same topic area.

Why do two systematic reviews on the same topic reach different conclusions?

With the increase in the number of systematic reviews, there is inevitably some duplication, especially in areas, which are 'interesting' or topical. Sometimes systematic reviews of the same topic area reach different conclusions, which can be confusing to practitioners. When this occurs, it is necessary to understand the methods behind the reviews, in order to understand why and how they differ. To illustrate, we examine the methods of two reviews of cranberry products for preventing urinary tract infections. While this preventive intervention may seem 'black and white' in its simplicity, we will show that the evidence on its effectiveness is subtly more complex.

Cranberries have been found to be a potentially useful preventative treatment as one of the active ingredients (proanthracyadins) can prevent bacteria (specifically *E. coli*) from adhering to the wall of the bladder. As urinary tract infections are a common problem, affecting specific population groups such as the elderly, people needing catheterization, and women, there is interest in preventative measures, which are acceptable and effective (and can potentially reduce antibiotic use). In 2012, two systematic reviews of cranberry juice for urinary tract infections were published. One was published in the Archives of Internal Medicine (AIM; Wang et al. 2012) and one was a Cochrane review (Jepson et al. 2012), published in the Cochrane Library. The two reviews had contradictory findings, both of which were widely reported in the media. The AIM review was published first (in July 2012) and newspapers ran the headlines such as 'Cranberry juice can protect against urine infections' (Roberts 2012). However, the Cochrane review, published three months later in October of 2012 reported that 'Cranberry juice 'won't prevent' bladder infections' (NHS Choices 2012). So, why did two high quality reviews come to such different conclusions (at least in the minds of the media)? The following are the typical sources of disagreement between structured reviews of a given body of evidence:

Differences in their quality

The methods that are used in systematic reviews aim to reduce bias and thus increase the extent to, which we can be confident in the findings (i.e. that the results are 'true'). A great deal of effort goes into searching for all the studies, applying inclusion criteria, assessing the quality of the primary studies, and making sure the conclusions match the results. As with primary research there are checklists for assessing the quality of systematic reviews; the link to one of these checklists, the AMSTAR checklist (which is easy to use yet thorough) is given in Appendix 2.

The author (RJ) has used AMSTAR to contrast the two reviews into whether cranberry juice prevents urinary tract infections (see Table 4.1); Cochrane: Jepson et al. (2012) and AIM: Wang et al. (2012)

One of the differences was that the Cochrane Review including both published *and* unpublished studies (so-called 'grey literature'). This resulted in more unpublished studies being included in the Cochrane review. This can be an important issue as unpublished studies are more likely to show little or no effect of an intervention. This is known as publication bias (see Box 4.3).

Differences in the included studies

Decisions about which studies should be included in a review and which ones should be excluded should be based on sound scientific principles. In both reviews, they appropriately included only the highest quality studies (RCTs). However, the Cochrane review included 24 studies, while the AIM included 13. The difference in number of trials was due to three main factors:

1. The Cochrane review included both published and unpublished studies (as already noted in Table 4.2).

2. The search dates for identifying studies were different. The Cochrane review searched up until July 2012 and included more studies published in 2010–2012 than the AIMs review (which searched for studies up until November 2011). The number of new studies published in 2012 indicates that this is a topic, which is of much interest to researchers, and producers of cranberry products.

3. The reviews had different inclusion and exclusion criteria for the interventions. The Cochrane paper included all studies that had a cranberry group compared with anything else (including other treatments such as antibiotics) whereas the AIMs review only included studies, which compared cranberry products with placebo or a non-treatment control.

Overall the AIM review did report similar results to the Cochrane review. The main difference was their decision to exclude one of the studies with women with recurrent UTIs from their meta-analysis. The exclusion of this single study (which showed that cranberries were *not* effective) was enough for the AIM analysis to demonstrate a statistically significant effect of the cranberries, i.e. an effect that was very unlikely to be due to chance alone. The Cochrane analysis (which included the study) demonstrated no statistically significant effect.

Table 4.1 A comparison of two reviews of the effectiveness of cranberry juice in preventing urinary tract infections, against AMSTAR criteria

Criterion	Cochrane	AIMs
1. *Was an 'a priori' design provided?* The research question and inclusion criteria should be established before the conduct of the review.	Yes	Can't answer
2. *Was there duplicate study selection and data extraction?* There should be at least two independent data extractors and a consensus procedure for disagreements should be in place.	Yes	Yes
3. *Was a comprehensive literature search performed?* At least two electronic sources should be searched. The report must include years and databases used (e.g. Central, EMBASE, and MEDLINE). Key words and/or MESH terms must be stated and where feasible the search strategy should be provided. All searches should be supplemented by consulting current contents, reviews, textbooks, specialized registers, or experts in the particular field of study, and by reviewing the references in the studies found.	Yes	Yes
4. *Was the status of publication (i.e. grey literature) used as an inclusion criterion?* The authors should state that they searched for reports regardless of their publication type. The authors should state whether or not they excluded any reports (from the systematic review), based on their publication status, language etc.	Yes	No
5. *Was a list of studies (included and excluded) provided?* A list of included and excluded studies should be provided.	Yes	No (excluded studies were not detailed)
6. *Were the characteristics of the included studies provided?* In an aggregated form such as a table, data from the original studies should be provided on the participants, interventions and outcomes. The ranges of characteristics in all the studies analysed, e.g. age, race, sex, relevant socioeconomic data, disease status, duration, severity, or other diseases should be reported.	Yes	Yes

Table 4.1 Continued

Criterion	Cochrane	AIMs
7. *Was the scientific quality of the included studies assessed and documented?* A priori methods of assessment should be provided (e.g. for effectiveness studies if the author(s) chose to include only randomized, double-blind, placebo-controlled studies, or allocation concealment as inclusion criteria); for other types of studies, alternative items will be relevant.	Yes	Yes
8. *Was the scientific quality of the included studies used appropriately in formulating conclusions?* The results of the methodological rigor and scientific quality should be considered in the analysis and the conclusions of the review, and explicitly stated in formulating recommendations.	Yes	Yes
9. *Were the methods used to combine the findings of studies appropriate?* For the pooled results, a test should be done to ensure the studies were combinable, to assess their homogeneity (i.e. Chi-squared test for homogeneity, I^2). If heterogeneity exists a random effects model should be used and/or the clinical appropriateness of combining should be taken into consideration (i.e. is it sensible to combine?).	Yes	Yes
10. *Was the likelihood of publication bias assessed?* An assessment of publication bias should include a combination of graphical aids (e.g. funnel plot, other available tests) and/ or statistical tests (e.g. Egger regression test).	Yes	Yes
11. *Was the conflict of interest stated?* Potential sources of support should be clearly acknowledged in both the systematic review and the included studies.	Yes	Can't answer

Source: data from Jepson, R.G. et al, 'Cranberries for preventing urinary tract infections', Copyright ©2012, advanced online publication, DOI: 10.1002/14651858.CD001321.pub5; and Wang, C.H. et al., 'Cranberry-containing products for prevention of urinary tract infections in susceptible populations: A systematic review and meta-analysis of randomized controlled trials', *Archives of Internal Medicine*, Volume 172, Issue 13, pp. 988–96, Copyright © 2012.

Box 4.3 Publication bias

Publication bias refers to the phenomenon whereby studies which show a positive result (e.g. that wonder drug 'marvellous' is better than placebo) are more likely to get published than those studies which show no effect ('marvellous' was no better than placebo). The subsequent over-representation of positive studies in systematic reviews may mean that the reviews are biased toward a positive result (e.g. showing an effect of 'marvellous' because more studies that showed an effect (than those that didn't) were published (not because it actually was any better). There are now methods available to determine whether there is a likelihood of a publication bias. In addition, many countries now have systems in place to ensure that all trials are registered (e.g. http://isrctn.org/). This registrations means that it is easier to identify those studies which haven't published their results.

Differences in the methods of analysis

Sometimes reviews use different approaches to analysing their included primary studies. For example, in a superb review of the effects of second-hand (environmental) tobacco smoke (ETS) on breast cancer (Miller et al. 2007) the authors separated for the first time those studies with high versus low quality assessments of ETS exposure. This innovation led to very different conclusions than prior reviews, which had not been convinced that there was evidence that ETS causes breast cancer.

What can we learn from the case study of cranberries and the prevention of urinary tract infections?

This case study of two reviews demonstrates how the decisions made when undertaking a systematic review (particularly in deciding, which studies to include, and how to analyse them) can have significant impacts for the results and conclusions on a topic, despite the process being transparent and open. Two sets of reviewers using similar methods (summarized in Table 4.2), but producing different conclusion.

So where does the 'truth' lie? In this case, the discrepancy in conclusions between the two reviews was primarily (but not exclusively) down to the inclusion or exclusion of a single study. If the effects of one single (in this case, small, but well designed) study can affect the results it probably means that although the overall effect size reached statistical significance, the clinical significance is likely to be very small (see Box 4.4).

Table 4.2 Methods for the two reviews

	Cochrane review	AIMs
Inclusion criteria	All randomized controlled trials (RCTs) or quasi-RCTs of cranberry products for the prevention of UTIs. Included comparisons with other treatments such as antibiotics	Randomized controlled trials (RCTs) comparing cranberry-containing products vs placebo or non-placebo control for prevention of UTI. Did not include studies of antibiotics
Databases searched	MEDLINE, EMBASE, the Cochrane Central Register of Controlled Trials (CENTRAL in The Cochrane Library) and the Internet [which retrieved a number of unpublished studies]	MEDLINE, EMBASE, and The Cochrane Controlled Trials Register (CCTR)
Date of last search	July 2012	November 2011
Total number of studies	24 (4,473 participants)	13 (1,616 participants)
Number evaluating cranberries vs placebo/control	23 [some studies included a cranberry group, another intervention group and a placebo/control group and so could be included]	13
Number included in a meta-analysis*	13 studies (2,462 participants)	10 (1,494 participants)

*The use of statistical methods to combine results of individual studies

Source: data from Jepson, R.G. et al, 'Cranberries for preventing urinary tract infections', Copyright © 2012, advanced online publication, DOI: 10.1002/14651858.CD001321.pub5; and Wang, C.H. et al., 'Cranberry-containing products for prevention of urinary tract infections in susceptible populations: A systematic review and meta-analysis of randomized controlled trials', *Archives of Internal Medicine*, Volume 172, Issue 13, pp. 988–96, Copyright © 2012.

The Cochrane review attempted to 'translate' the finding of the review into practice (e.g. make a judgement about effectiveness rather than just efficacy (Box 4.1)). When making their conclusions and recommendations, the Cochrane researchers took the following into account to understand what might happen if cranberry products were used in the real world:

Box 4.4 Statistical versus clinical significance

To be clinically significant, an intervention needs to substantially change an outcome to a degree that matters from a clinician's or patient's perspective. Statistically significant changes, however, can be observed with trivial (small) changes in important outcomes, if the study has a large enough sample size. Large studies can find statistically significant effects that are not clinically important, and small studies may find differences which are potentially clinically important, but not statistically significant (Hennekens et al. 1987).

1. *The natural history of UTIs.* Cranberry products were most beneficial to women who had *recurrent* UTIs. The natural history of the disease in women who have recurrent UTI is that they tend to cluster, so a woman may have two or three UTIs in a short period of time and then not have any more for a considerable length of time. This means that, not only is it difficult to know how many UTIs could have been prevented, it is also difficult to estimate the length of time a woman would need to take cranberry products in order to prevent a single UTI: one year? 2 years?

2. *The 'potency' of cranberry products: relevance to benefits and harms.* The second issue is the potency of cranberry products. The potency or effect of the active ingredient in cranberries only lasts for 10 hours in its juice form, so two doses (glasses of cranberry juice) per day at least are needed to provide full 24 hour protection. Other products such as capsules and tablets may be more acceptable, but there is still work to be undertaken to ensure that the potency in the dried form is equivalent to that in the juice.

3. *Adherence to the intervention.* Two glasses of cranberry juice every day, more or less indefinitely, is quite a commitment for a preventative measure, and it is also calorific and can be expensive to buy. Some women may be willing to commit to drinking this amount for an indeterminate amount of time (which will maximize its effectiveness), but others may not adhere to such a regimen (thereby making it less effective).

This example illustrates two separate, but important points. Firstly, evidence on efficacy demonstrated in clinical trials is not enough to make public health decisions. We need to understand the natural history of the disease or condition, the nature of the intervention and the context in which it operates. Urinary tract infections have a fairly simple causal pathway (the bladder is the host, the bacteria is the agent), and the cranberry product is used to interrupt this causal pathway (by preventing the bacteria from adhering to the wall of the bladder). It has some sound evidence of effect, but this is unlikely to translate into an effective intervention for women because of the difficulties and adverse effects of implementation (in this case drinking the product) and uncertainty as to the dose and the duration of the intervention. Secondly, the clinically significant effectiveness of an intervention is different from the statistical significance (see Box 4.4). In this instance, the addition of a single study made one set of reviewers find a statistically significant effect *overall*, but it had very little clinical significance. Evidence based guidelines can help with deciding what is clinically significant.

Evidence-based guidelines

Evidence-based guidance takes into account *both* the research evidence and the views of stakeholders. Several national bodies undertake guideline development including the Canadian Task Force on Preventive Health Care (n.d.), the US Preventive Services Task Force (2015) and the NICE: National Institute for Health and Care Excellence (2014) in England and Wales. NICE are internationally recognized for the way in, which they develop their recommendations, a rigorous process that is centred on using the best available evidence and includes the views of experts, patients, carers, and industry. NICE guidance is created by independent and unbiased advisory committees.

In 2005, NICE was asked to develop guidance on behaviour change. The process was open and transparent, and went through a rigorous process (see Table 4.3). Six evidence-based reviews were commissioned, and other cost-effectiveness reviews were undertaken in-house by NICE staff. What is interesting about this guidance is that, although the guideline developers (known as the Programme Development Group or PDG) had a plethora of research evidence available to them, they did not use it to guide people towards specific interventions (e.g. mass media, motivational techniques). Instead they opted to make a series of 'principles' including:

♦ Base interventions on a proper assessment of the target group.

♦ Work with other organizations and the community itself.

♦ Build on the skills and knowledge that already exists in the community.

♦ Take account of, and resolve problems that prevent people changing their behaviour (for example, the costs involved in taking part in exercise programmes, or buying fresh fruit and vegetables, or lack of knowledge about how to make changes).

Table 4.3 Developing guidance on behaviour change: the principles for effective interventions*

Steps	Further description
Topic selected	For NICE by Department of Health (for England and Wales) to develop public health programme guidance on supporting knowledge, attitude, and behaviour change.
Stakeholders register interest	Stakeholders included practitioners, NHS boards, professional bodies, relevant industries, charities, lay public, and academic institutions
Scope prepared	*Key question*: What are the most appropriate generic and specific interventions to support attitude and behaviour change at population and community levels? A committee (the Programme Development Group or PDG) is convened.
Evidence reviewed	◆ Six reviews undertaken • *Review 1*: effectiveness of interventions for six health-related behaviours.[†] • *Review 2*: effectiveness of road-safety and pro-environmental interventions. • *Review 3*: resilience, coping and salutogenic approaches. • *Review 4*: use of theories of health behaviour to study and predict health-related behaviour change. • *Review 5*: social and cultural context on the effectiveness of health behaviour change interventions in relation to diet, exercise, and smoking cessation, • *Review 6*: social marketing, Plus a cost-effectiveness review undertaken internally by NICE
Call for evidence and draft guidance prepared	At its first meetings, the PDG considered the evidence of effectiveness and cost-effectiveness and theoretical and methodological evidence. Initially, discussions focused on the evidence outlined in the reviews. The PDG also considered evidence on cost-effectiveness, evidence from fieldwork, additional review material and a range of theoretical and methodological approaches. The PDG considered comments from stakeholders and the results from fieldwork to determine: whether there was sufficient evidence (in terms of quantity, quality and applicability) to form a judgement or whether, on balance, the evidence demonstrates that the intervention is effective or ineffective, or whether it is equivocal where there is an effect, the typical size of effect. The PDG developed draft recommendations through informal consensus, based on the theoretical ideas that informed its view of behaviour, and the degree to which the available effectiveness evidence could support these ideas.

Table 4.3 Continued

Steps	Further description
Consultation on the draft guidance	The draft guidance, including the recommendations, was released for consultation in April 2007.
Fieldwork carried out	Qualitative interviews with 97 individuals, either in small groups or individually, across 30 sites. Participants included representatives from the DH, other government departments and arm's length bodies, directors of public health in Primary Care Trusts and strategic health authorities, public health advisers, health promotion staff and NHS practitioners, community-based school nurses, health trainers; and commissioners, service providers and practitioners working in local and national charities.
Final guidance produced and issued	The guidance was signed off by the NICE Guidance Executive in September 2007.

*All relevant documents can be access here: http://www.nice.org.uk/guidance/index.jsp?action=byId&o=11675&history=t#stakeholders

† Updated review http://www.biomedcentral.com/1471-2458/10/538/

National Institute for Health and Clinical Excellence (2007). Adapted from *PH 6 Behaviour change: general approaches*. London: NICE. Available at: www.nice.org.uk/PH6. Reproduced with permission. Information accurate at time of press. For up-to-date guidance please visit www.nice.org.uk

- ◆ Base all interventions on evidence of what works.
- ◆ Train staff to help people change their behaviour.
- ◆ Evaluate all interventions.

Table 4.3 shows how guidance is developed and the role of research evidence.

Decision support tool

Evidence assessment—1A, B, and C.

Considering the individual, community, or population perspectives—1, 3, and 4.

Considering your personal perspective.

Quiz

Readers interested in more detail about the science of 'evidence synthesis' are referred to in the writings of J. P. Ioannidis (2005) concerning the fundamental reasons that so much of the published literature on most health questions is (to use his word) 'wrong' or, at least, methodologically flawed. If the reader wants to demonstrate for him/herself just how challenging it is to find replicable sets of studies for a given structured review, try comparing all the high-quality studies identified on a controversial question in prevention, e.g. mammography for detecting early breast cancer. Compare two authoritative and widely cited structured reviews published about the same time (e.g. Independent UK Panel on Breast Cancer Screening 2012; US Preventive Services Task Force 2009b), while excluding any primary studies published after the first review appeared.

Chapter 5

Causation and prevention in populations versus individuals

Obesity: why has it increased so rapidly and widely?

The descriptive facts of the 'outbreak' of obesity (and its less severe manifestation, 'overweight'[10]) are widely known and agreed upon. Across many high-income countries, we have decades-long time series on trends in weight for height at the population level—often summarized as Body Mass Index (BMI) (weight in kilograms, divided by height in metres squared). These time series show clearly that a dramatic increase in BMI began to happen in the 1980s, initially in the USA. The epidemic then spread much more widely, as it accelerated over the next ten to twenty years. More human beings became heavier than is healthy, than has ever been seen in recorded history. Leading the pack, with earlier and more extensive spread of the epidemic, have been the Americas, where over two-thirds of adults are now obese or overweight, and more than one in three children (Butland et al. 2007; Finucane et al. 2011). However, as time has gone on, even countries that appeared to be protected initially from this dramatic shift (such as parts of the Mediterranean region), presumably shielded by certain features of their traditional cultures and cuisines (Chapter 6) have also now experienced major increases in body weight. Many middle-income countries have recently seen large increases in body weight among their wealthier citizens, especially in urban areas. One country, Mexico, has shot up in the international rankings of obesity prevalence within a much shorter time (just over a decade), ending up as the second-most-affected country in the world, after the USA, which is of course, its next door neighbour, so that both countries are subject to similar trade agreements and food marketing practices, as well as cultural trends.

While there is no absolute scientific agreement as to what drove this pandemic, and keeps driving it today, one thing is certain: it could not be genetic factors acting by themselves. Human and animal populations' genetic compositions cannot change that rapidly, barring massive lethal epidemics. However the obesity pandemic has arisen first and fastest in some of the world's previously healthiest populations, with very low (and still declining) death rates. Although most experts are predicting that the pandemic itself may change that rosy picture within the next few decades. That is because the serious chronic diseases arising from long-term obesity, e.g. type 2 diabetes, coronary heart disease, stroke, osteoarthritis, and a number of different cancers, take some decades to develop and lead to lethal complications (Butland et al. 2007). With genetics essentially 'held constant' over such a short period of history, public health experts agree that the principal drivers of this pandemic must lie in the environment around us, both physical and cultural. And the prevailing opinion is that the main drivers of this change were shifts in our culture, together with the 'built environment' designed and used by mankind, as well as our food production and marketing, particularly as they affect the caloric content of our food, our eating habits, and physical activity patterns (Butland et al. 2007).

This is not to say that the individuals most affected by this pandemic are in any sense a random sample of the populations affected. Indeed, many epidemiological and laboratory science studies have identified both genetic and biological markers of risk, as well as personal and family-level risk factors that determine, which individuals are more likely to develop the greatest degree of overweight, and at what age, *under a given set of 'obesogenic' environmental influences* (Butland et al. 2007). However, several countries now have reached the point where more of their populations are overweight than of normal weight, typically involving more than a tripling of rates of obesity seen in the same countries before 1980. This suggests that profound 'upstream' forces must have been operating to drive this 'tsunami' of health risk over less than four decades, forces involving aspects of mass culture that have now affected the majority of persons in these entire populations. In fact, there is a rapidly growing scientific literature about 'obesogenic' cultural and physical environments, which seem capable, at least in the worst affected societies, such as the USA of making all, but a minority of persons in *virtually any* society overweight by mid-life, sparing only those individuals with very strong personal eating and exercise habits that confer 'resistance' to obesogenic influences.

There are a small number of researchers who continue to search for less obvious factors, which may have precipitated the rather sudden onset of the obesity pandemic. One should not dismiss the possibility that these investigators will eventually identify a completely exogenous biological driver of what has happened to hundreds of millions of people in one generation. For example, in a novel hypothesis published in 2013, a group of infectious disease biologists suggested that the culprit may have been accumulation in our environment, and in our bodies, of antibiotics (Riley et al. 2013; Schulz et al. 2014). These drugs are widely used in both modern animal husbandry (somewhat ironically, to promote more rapid weight gain, as well as to control disease) and in modern medical practice (where they are well documented to be overused). Their paper implicates changes in the complex, and largely unstudied, bacterial flora of our mouths, stomachs, and intestinal systems. Changes caused by ubiquitous antibiotic exposure since birth, as the key factor initiating the obesity pandemic. Further research will likely confirm or refute this hypothesis.

Until then, public health experts and medical practitioners around the world have only two basic tools for preventing[11] the further development of overweight in persons (especially children) not yet affected: decreasing their calorie intake; and/or increasing their physical activity/reducing their sedentary behaviour to burn off more calories. Unfortunately, both involve substantial behaviour change, sustained over years, and are difficult to achieve in the midst of todays powerfully obesogenic environments and cultures (National Institute for Health and Clinical Excellence 2006b).

To be more specific, recent epidemiological studies have pointed to two underlying drivers of this pandemic, which appear to be replicated in each country in the years leading up to the first signs of major increases in body weight:

1. The widespread adoption of modern food manufacturing and marketing, involving the production, wide distribution and mass-consumption of high-calorie-density foods such as sugared beverages and snacks, as well as deep-fried 'fast foods', replacing more traditional foods cooked at home, and typically of lower calorie density.

2. A decline in walking and high-exertion physical activity, formerly required for transport and work (paid, as well as unpaid, in the home.) That decline is linked to the widespread adoption of motorized transport, often closely associated with urbanization, as well as less physically demanding jobs, replacing age-old patterns of traditional human body use (Lang and Rayner 2007).

How is it that these 'upstream determinants' of the global obesity pandemic, are so powerful that they can convert more than half of a country's population to overweight persons, and more than a quarter of those populations into obese patients, requiring aggressive medical treatment to reduce imminent health risks, within a few decades? Most experts believe that these upstream *societal obesogenic* forces' have completely overwhelmed affected *individuals'* personal protective factors (both genetic, as well as lifetime experiences and exposures, beginning with prolonged and exclusive breast-feeding exposure, and healthy family eating habits as children (Mooney et al. 2015; Wang et al. 2008)). On the other hand, it is also true that the biological history of human beings is such that we store excess ingested energy for times of famine, it is only in the modern era of lifelong excess caloric intake that this has become unhealthy.

The obesity pandemic is a clear example of one of the most insightful statements ever made by an epidemiologist about two parallel processes in chronic disease causation, the British cardiovascular expert Geoffrey Rose:

> The determinants of incidence [disease occurrence in populations] are not necessarily the same as the causes of [individual] cases (Rose 1985, p. 35).

To illustrate in another way what Rose meant by this statement, one can perform a thought experiment about smoking. Imagine a society where everyone smoked regularly, from the end of childhood, until death. In epidemiological studies of such a society's lung cancer cases, comparing them with controls without lung cancer, no direct effect of smoking could be observed, simply because there are no 'unexposed' persons (i.e. non-smokers) in the population. The development of lung cancer, which is known to occur in less than 10% of smokers in our world (where less than 50% of most adult populations now smoke) would instead be found to be related to patterns of lifelong nutrition, and individual genetic make-up (Rothman et al. 2008). In a similar way, once a clear majority of a whole society becomes overweight or obese, through the ubiquitous effects of an obesogenic environment and culture, epidemiological studies of obesity cases within that society, compared to normal-weight controls, will tend to identify largely *individual-level risk factors* such as infant and child nutrition, in the context of family eating and exercising habits, and adults' personal physical activity and nutritional patterns. One can only study, using classical epidemiological study designs at the level of the individual (e.g. cohort and case control studies) the influence of causal factors that vary in their exposure levels within a given study population (Rothman et al. 2008).

It follows that a holistic approach to obesity prevention, given that entire societies' patterns of obesogenic risk-factor exposure have changed substantially within half of one average human lifespan, needs to consider *both* the 'causes of cases' (at the individual level) and the 'causes of incidence' (at the population level). More pointedly, successful prevention and control of the current pandemic of overweight and obesity, wherever it is firmly established, can hardly be feasible purely through *individual-level* medical care, whether it be nutritional and activity counselling and behaviour-change methods, or more radical treatments for the more severely affected. Not only would the costs of such individualized, long-term medical care for so many affected patients (especially in the USA, Mexico, and the UK) bankrupt even the richest nation. In addition, the ongoing production of new cases, amongst children and youth in each fresh generation, would not be effectively stemmed by focusing on the severe, late-stage cases in which aggressive (and expensive) treatments are most cost-effective. Furthermore, to prevent those new cases, *primary and secondary prevention* alone will not be enough, if it is targeted only at the individual. Rather, *primordial* preventive measures (Chapter 2), at the level of the entire culture and environment, affecting the whole population, will have to be enacted, tackling the upstream drivers that determine the disordered patterns of nutrition and activity that caused the emergence of the pandemic in the first place.

The insight quoted above led Rose to its corollary: that **both** *upstream/ entire-population-level exposures to chronic disease risk factors, as well as more downstream and intensive treatments, targeted at the individual level in fully developed, more severe cases, are required in order to optimally control most chronic diseases.* Indeed, Rose offered up examples of many risk factors for chronic conditions, requiring this dual approach to prevention and control. [He was particularly knowledgeable about cardiovascular risk factors and disease, and so focused on examples such as hypertension (high blood pressure), high blood cholesterol levels, and increased blood glucose (sugar) levels that signal early diabetes (Rose 2008)].

Figure 5.1 illustrates Rose's idea schematically, showing how the 'bell curve' of any traditional hunter-gather or early agrarian society's population distributions of BMI (depicted at the left side of the graph) have been shifted to

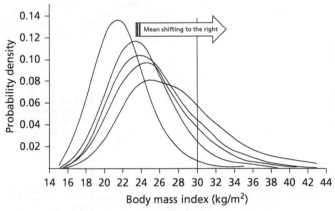

Fig. 5.1 Rose's example of entire population distributions of BMI around the World—the shifting distributions of body mass index of five population groups of men and women aged 20–59 years derived from 52 surveys in 32 countries.

Adapted from Rose, G., *The strategy of preventive medicine, Revised edition*, Figure 5.2b, p. 93, Oxford University Press, Oxford, UK, Copyright © 2008, by permission of Oxford University Press.

the right (due to much higher BMI levels throughout the population, eventually affecting all, but the small minority of 'resistantly thin' persons in today's worst-affected societies). For those with established obesity, to the right of the vertical line under the right 'tail' of these distributions, intensive (and expensive) medical treatment is both cost-effective and ethically mandated. However, the much more numerous, but less severely affected persons who are merely overweight and not yet obese, those sitting more towards the middle of the BMI distributions, within the populations of modern, obesogenic environments and cultures, who have only modestly elevated BMI levels, would be more appropriately managed by a combination of primordial (societal-level) and tertiary (individual-level) *prevention*, rather than intensive treatment. The goal of such preventive programmes and policies would obviously be to reduce these moderately affected persons' chances of progressing to higher BMI levels, thus preventing future obesity-related disease. This will require, as virtually all authoritative reviews of the question have concluded (Lang and Rayner 2007) vigorous population-level measures targeting the entire society—such as taxes on high-energy-density food and drink, and active transportation policies designed to incentivize physical activity by environmental re-design and motorized transport taxation/pricing (National Institute for Health and Clinical Excellence 2006b). These two approaches to prevention and control of obesity are schematically depicted in Figure 5.2.

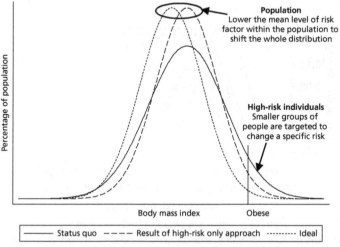

Fig. 5.2 Rose's two complementary approaches to preventing chronic disease: the example of obesity.

Adapted from Rose, G., *The strategy of preventive medicine, Revised edition*, Figure 6.5, p. 108, Oxford University Press, Oxford, UK, Copyright © 1992, by permission of Oxford University Press.

To reiterate, neither of these two approaches to chronic disease prevention and control is adequate in and of itself to properly deal with the pandemic, and one is not 'better' than the other, they are mutually complementary and synergistic. Therefore, when the need for both approaches is not recognized, problems arise in developing evidence-based health policy and planning likely to successfully address the pandemic. For example, we sometimes read recommendations from special interest groups, such as private weight-loss clinics, who would have us, believe that everyone with even a minor/early weight problem should be clinically assessed and intensively treated as individual, medicalized patients. Often unstated, but clearly implied in such recommendations is that such intensive treatments will have to be continued more or less indefinitely, given that higher levels of overweight tend to be a relapsing condition, requiring years to decades of persistent treatment, especially within the adverse context of obesogenic cultures and environments. This approach would no doubt ensure an endless queue of patients for these clinic entrepreneurs, but lead to an unsustainable medical bill for society. Furthermore, this approach might well not even achieve adequate weight control among many of those treated, at least with current behavioural change treatments, which tend to have relatively high drop-out rates and unimpressive long-term outcomes, although the widely available Counterweight programme in the UK is a positive exception (McCombie et al. 2012).

Perhaps most important of all, the medicalization of overweight as entirely an individually-based behavioural problem, characterized as arising from abnormal psychological, behavioural and physiological processes inside a person, is often accompanied by a virtual denial of the importance of upstream societal, obesogenic, forces in the causal process. Yet the extraordinary speed and extent of the modern pandemic's spread, in just over three decades, strongly suggests that intra-personal processes alone could not be the whole cause of what has happened, the innate psychology and physiology of individual human beings is unlikely to have changed that much, over such a short period. Consequently, public health authorities are of the unanimous view that any effective and sustainable response to the pandemic must involve societal-level policies and programmes that can shift the key upstream drivers, factors altering an entire population's behavioural patterns around eating and physical activity.

Worrisomely, public health authorities note that in some countries the pandemic has not yet fully 'exhausted the susceptible individuals', the usual mechanism by which infectious disease epidemics run their course and peter out (Wang et al. 2008). Thus, in the USA for example, even the sky-high rates of child obesity of 13 years earlier continued to rise, to reach 17% of all American children by 2012 (Skinner and Skelton 2014). Fortunately, increasing research evidence suggests that those unhealthy behavioural patterns can be effectively and efficiently changed by government policies and programmes, which alter the incentives and disincentives for engaging in them: price, marketing practices, as well as availability of and access to alternatives to unhealthy foods and activity patterns (Stuckler et al. 2012). Such changes are unlikely to occur spontaneously, especially in societies with laissez-fair economic policies, since current patterns of marketing for unhealthy food and drink, and non-physically active past-times (such as those involving watching screens) turn out to be very profitable for sellers, and enjoyable for consumers. That is why more critical public health experts are increasingly insisting on legislation and regulation to change the marketing, production, and distribution practices of the relevant industries (Brownell and Warner 2009; Lang and Rayner 2007; Moodie et al. 2013; Mooney et al. 2015).

A corollary of Rose's prevention insights: evaluating the success of population-level preventive interventions often requires different scientific methods

Moving on from understanding the drivers of the obesity pandemic to considering some potentially effective public health policy and programme responses to it, we need to reconsider the question addressed in Chapter 3, concerning how one can best establish the success or failure of preventive measures. There we were concerned with prevention directed at individuals, such as clinically delivered dietary or lifestyle advice, vaccines to prevent infectious diseases (and related cancers, e.g. HPV infection, the cause of almost all cases of cancer of the cervix), as well as prescribed supplements and drugs. In that chapter, we focused on the importance of randomized controlled trials (RCTs) for scientifically establishing in a robust way that such preventive measures, directed at individuals, are effective, in terms of actually reducing the future risk of undesirable health outcomes, without unreasonable risks. However, for preventive policies and programmes directed at entire communities or societies (i.e. populations) it is often logistically impossible, or even unethical, to randomize study subjects to 'intervention' and 'control' groups in an RCT. Fortunately, public health researchers can utilize other study designs to evaluate the success of preventive interventions designs, which have been on the ascendancy recently, as more and more social scientists and economists influence public health thinking, with their long history of using such non-randomized evaluative methods for interventions at the population level (Craig et al. 2011; Des Jarlais et al. 2004; Sanson-Fisher et al. 2014).

The examples cited below show the kinds of circumstances, and public health preventive interventions, which frequently cannot be evaluated using an

RCT design. Listed below are three broad categories of circumstances wherein it is difficult or impossible to use RCT evaluations for preventive interventions:

1. Circumstances *where the preventive intervention cannot be randomized to individual subjects because it would not be ethical to do so*, for example randomizing pregnant women to breastfeed or formula-feed; the evidence in favour of breast feeding is now so compelling, except in very special medical circumstances, that one could not, quite rightly, convince a Human Subjects (Ethical) Review Board, the final arbiters of what research is allowed in all universities and public sector institutions, that such a study is ethical.

2. Circumstances *where the preventive intervention can only be delivered to an entire community/population, as opposed to individuals*, because of its essential nature—for example, the fluoridation of public water supplies to prevent dental caries (tooth decay); while individuals can be given fluoride supplements in various forms, including having fluoride painted on their teeth, that is not the same as fluoridating an entire public water supply. Fluoridation requires preventive trials of precisely that intervention, in order to be sure that enough fluoride is ingested by the target population (especially children) to reduce caries development, without causing the signs of excessive fluoride dosing (an easily diagnosed dental and bone condition called fluorosis). See Box 5.1 for the details of a famous evaluation of this intervention. This evaluation challenge also applies to virtually all legislative and regulatory interventions, including taxes, subsides and marketing restrictions, such as those currently under consideration or actually being deployed for unhealthy lifestyle exposures such as tobacco, excessive alcohol, sugared beverages, trans-fats in foods, etc.

3. Circumstances *where the intervention could be randomized to groups of subjects,* randomized as groups, through a technique called 'cluster randomization' (Sanson-Fisher et al. 2014), *but the design entails logistics and costs that are prohibitive*—for example, an RCT of paying pregnant women to stop smoking would be difficult to implement within any one clinical setting, where waiting room and neighbourhood conversations are likely to make it known who is and who is not receiving these extra payments, potentially leading to jealousies and complaints. Using geographically separated antenatal clinics, in which some women are paid and others are not, might be feasible, but the only way to ensure that the two groups of clinics' patients are fully comparable on factors that might influence the outcome is to randomize a rather large number of entire antenatal clinic clienteles to each arm of the trial, a number determined in part by how homogeneous all the clinics are across these factors. Yet, even if such detailed planning statistics are locally available before conducting such a study, onerous sample-sizes may be required for the trial, as well as significant logistic challenges.

Box 5.1 Some examples of public health interventions evaluated by non-RCT designs

Community water supply fluoridation trial (North America, 1960s and later)

More than 40 years ago, there was ample animal and laboratory science to suggest that carefully controlled addition of fluoride to community water supplies would reduce dental caries (still the commonest dental condition), while not causing fluorosis or other manifestations of fluoride poisoning. To prove that, an ingenious study was designed involving three pairs of North American cities with single public water supplies, with each pair matched on particular characteristics which might impact the health benefits and risks of fluoridation (baseline dental health, based on surveys, as well as baseline naturally occurring levels of fluoride in the local water, although all six communities had natural fluoride levels too low for dental protection). Within each pair of cities, one had its water fluoridated, and one did not. Over some years of follow-up, careful repeat dental examinations of young people in each community revealed an impressive 50% reduction in the onset of new dental caries cases, and no evidence of fluorosis or other harm. This non-RCT evidence was particularly convincing because:

◆ It was replicated in each of the three pairs of cities, with very homogeneous results

◆ There were, and are today, no other major factors likely to change during the trial that are known to influence dental caries development so powerfully, e.g. dental care practices and dietary intake of sugary foods was not manipulated by the investigators and did not appear to change in any way that could have affected the trial's observed results.

For further information see Horowitz (1996).

Smoke free legislation's effects on hospitalisations for acute coronary syndrome (Scotland, 2006)

This widely praised study is an example of a 'natural experiment' with time-series of before- and after-intervention measures of the primary outcome (Scottish hospitalizations for acute coronary syndrome (ACS)), as well as of the same outcomes, identically-timed, for the English population, where no ban on smoking in public places occurred. Indeed, a key element in this elegant study's design is that there was a very comparable 'control' population right across the border with England, which had not yet implemented such smoking legislation (Craig et al. 2011). Those data clearly showed no such major reduction in ACS admissions to hospital during the period when they dropped by nearly 20% in Scotland, starting within weeks of the ban, thereby making it very unlikely that some other contemporaneous factor, such as unusual weather, or circulating influenza strain or other infection, or altered patterns of medical care, was responsible for the major health benefits documented after the legislation was enacted in Scotland. Another methodological strength of this study was that the critical intermediary variable, exposure to second-hand smoke (SHS) in the population before and after the ban, was carefully measured. That analysis showed a 90% reduction in SHS exposure in bar workers, as determined by salivary cotinine levels, and a 40% reduction in representative samples of adults and children in the general population. See Pell et al. (2008) for further information.

Paying Indian women to give birth in a health facility, the abolition of GP fund-holding in the UK, and evaluation of the English Sure-Start Early Childhood Education Initiative

These published studies are thoroughly described by Craig et al. (2011) in their comprehensive guidance on conducting non-RCT 'natural experiment' evaluations of public health interventions (or indeed any deliberate interventions delivered at the population level). In each case a particular design 'trick' was used:

♦ Creating credible control groups of subjects who did not receive the intervention, usually for more or less 'random' reasons (e.g. the children in the Sure Start Evaluation who lived in counties just above and just below the income-distribution cut-offs for programme eligibility) – the 'regression discontinuity design'.

♦ Utilizing extensive additional information to create 'matched' individuals in the intervention and control groups, in terms of multiple factors likely to influence the study's primary outcome, as a constructed control group (the Indian birth-facility study) – the 'propensity score approach'.

+ Using time-series of outcomes before and after the intervention in both treatment and control groups, to be able—using methods borrowed from econometrics, such as 'difference in differences analysis' to adjust for previous discrepancies in time-trends in the two groups (the evaluation of the Abolition of GP Fund-holding.)

In the last case the authors also analysed outcome not likely to be affected by the intervention—as a kind of 'instrumental variable' to check that other changes in the treatment and control practices were not going on during the intervention period.

Source: data from Craig, P. et al., *Developing and evaluating complex interventions: new guidance*, Medical Research Council, London, UK, Copyright © 2008, available from http://www.mrc.ac.uk/documents/pdf/developing-and-evaluating-complex-interventions/

Fortunately, in these situations where RCTs are either impossible or very difficult to use for robustly evaluating preventive interventions at the population level, researchers have a number of alternative study designs at their disposal, which are generally termed 'quasi-experimental' or 'observational' studies. A detailed discussion of the pros and cons of each of them is beyond the scope of this book: the reader is referred to recent helpful reviews (Craig et al. 2011; Sanson-Fisher et al. 2014). Box 5.1 provides a number of specific examples of such studies that have yielded relatively conclusive results that have stood the test of time.

What can the reader do for him/herself to ensure that such non-RCT evidence of preventive effectiveness passes muster, scientifically speaking? The best approach is to use a widely accepted, peer-reviewed checklist of criteria for both study design and analysis, and for accurate and full reporting, of such evaluations. An example of the former, developed by our colleague Professor Sally Haw of the University of Stirling a few years ago, and taught by the authors on several occasions since, is a Critical Appraisal checklist for Non-RCT (Quasi-Experimental) Evaluations of Intervention Effectiveness.

One last word is necessary in order to help the reader deal with some historical writing in this field, which has sometimes had a rancorous tone. In the recent history of epidemiology, there have been widely respected scientific voices calling for, and in some cases practically insisting on, the use of RCTs for evaluating the effectiveness of virtually all health interventions, on the grounds of their superior 'internal validity' (i.e. their ability to rule out spurious differences in trial outcomes due to confounding factors, even unknown ones, that differ between the intervention and control groups, through randomization.)

These voices have typically come from experts in 'clinical epidemiology', a branch of the discipline concerned with studies of what happens to, and what is done to, patients under medical care as individuals. In such circumstances, there is almost always a feasible and ethical way to randomize individual patients to receive a new intervention or not, and so RCTs are indeed the gold standard for effectiveness evaluation in clinical studies. However, in public health practice, where the entire community/population is typically being intervened upon, usually to prevent future illness or injury, the examples provided illustrate how commonly RCTs are either infeasible or unethical, thus requiring researchers evaluating such programmes and policies to creatively utilize novel quasi-experimental and observational study designs instead, such as those described.

Decision support tool

Evidence assessment—2C and E.

Considering the individual, community or population perspectives—3.

Considering your personal perspective.

Quiz

Apply the checklist below to the study described (Box 5.1) by Pell et al. (2008) of the effects on hospitalizations for acute coronary syndrome (ACS—'heart attack') of Scotland's implementation of smoke-free legislation in 2006, banning smoking in public places. Suggested model answers are available in Appendix 3.

1. **Did the study ask a clearly focused question?**
   Were the population, intervention, and outcomes clearly defined?
2. **Was a quasi-experimental design appropriate?**
   Could an RCT have been conducted to assess the impact of the intervention under study?
3. **What are the key features of the quasi-experimental design used in this study?**
   - What was the study design?
   - What were the primary outcome measures?
   - What were the secondary outcome measures?
   - How were sub-groups defined in the intervention group?
   - What other study designs have been used elsewhere to address this question?

4. **Were the analyses appropriate and clearly presented?**
5. **Are the results clearly presented?**
   - Patients included in the study.
   - Primary outcomes.
   - Secondary outcomes.
6. **Is the interpretation of findings appropriate?**
   - Are the findings biologically plausibility?
   - Are the findings consistent with the proposed mechanisms of the legislation?
   - Is there any evidence of selection bias?
   - Is there any evidence of loss to follow-up or differential follow up?
   - Are the control groups and their outcome measures appropriate?
   - Are alternative explanations of findings ruled out?

Acknowledgments

Chapter 5 quiz questions reproduced courtesy of Sally Haw, Professor of Public and Population Health, University of Stirling, UK.

Chapter 6

How simple advice can sometimes be wrong—the case of 'healthy diets'

How science establishes the healthiness of foods

In Chapter 3, the authors pointed out how epidemiology combines with the basic laboratory sciences to build up a body of evidence that any 'exposure' likely does or does not cause a specific health effect, primarily by conducting cohort (and in some cases, case-control) studies. The reader will remember that such epidemiological studies make up only one part of the overall evidence base for asserting that an exposure, such as a food eaten regularly, leads to or protects from a specific disease, by showing that the exposure and outcome are statistically associated, preferably with a moderate to high relative risk (RR), and ideally with a clear dose-response relationship between exposure intensity ('dose') and the RR of the outcome. When enough high-quality studies of this kind have met these purely epidemiological criteria for causation, then systematic reviews of other sorts of evidence, typically from animal and other laboratory studies are also taken into consideration, to see whether the other causation criteria listed in Box 3.1 are met.

Dietary studies of disease causation are no different in principle from studies of non-dietary exposures. Many excellent dietary cohort studies have been conducted in the last half century, leading to robust findings widely replicated, that are the basis for many of the world's dietary guidelines (Public Health England 2015; US Department of Agriculture and US Department of Health and Human Service 2015). However, there are significant scientific challenges to both designing and conducting such diet and disease studies properly, and in interpreting the results to derive sound dietary advice for the general population. Listed in Box 6.1, are the major potential sources of disagreement, and sometimes frank error, in nutritional

Box 6.1 Common sources of error and disagreement in nutritional epidemiology

Determining precisely what a person eats, over the many years that are typically involved in the causal pathway between diet and major 'chronic' disease, is fraught with challenges

Most people do not remember precisely what they have eaten for more than a few days, but asking them to keep a detailed diary of all that they eat, for longer than a few days, is difficult for most study subjects to comply with. This situation leads to a great deal of 'measurement error' in the assessment of long-term dietary patterns at the individual level. Such error frequently obscures associations, especially for foods eaten infrequently (because one would have to keep a diary for a long time to capture when they are eaten) and also those eaten very frequently (because they are so much a staple in an individual's diet that precise amounts consumed can be easily mis-stated). And then there are 'halo effects' wherein respondents are reluctant to report unhealthy or excessive patterns of consumption, tending to convert them into healthier alternative reports, perhaps even subconsciously in some cases.

Ensuring that persons who eat in unusual ways, compared to most people in their cultural setting, are not different in some other way that may actually be contributing to the observed unhealthy or protective effect on a disease outcome, is never easy

The more of an 'outlier' such persons with unusual dietary habits are, the more likely it is that other aspects of their diet, lifestyle or other personal habits are the underlying reason for observing an association between eating a particularly unusual food, or unusual quantities of a local staple, and developing a disease. In short, outlier dietary exposures are often confounded by other subtle factors which are not necessarily known, let alone measurable with accuracy, so they may not be fully taken account of in multivariate statistical analyses.

Sometimes the laboratory science needed to be sure whether a given food contains precisely the same chemical compounds as another food, implicated in disease causation, lags behind the epidemiological studies

This situation can lead to the scientific promulgation of wrongful advice about that food, which is only cleared up later when more sophisticated chemical analyses reveals that the foods in question are actually quite different in composition than previously thought, in ways that importantly affect how healthy they are.

Finally, there is a serious statistical hazard associated with cohort or case-control studies that collect data from thousands of human subjects, about their consumption levels for dozens to hundreds of types of food (using a standard 'food frequency questionnaire') and then analyse those consumption levels against many different disease outcomes

The extensive searching for associations between specific foods and specific diseases leads to a statistical challenge: the chances that some associations found will be due to chance alone—and therefore represent 'false positive' findings—is greatly increased, and is not entirely reduced by standard adjustments to the analysis for '*multiple hypothesis testing*' (Rothman et al. 2008). As a result, single nutritional epidemiological studies of new associations between eating patterns and diseases, tend to be over-interpreted. Considering such studies in isolation, without careful consideration of the results of other studies of the same association (and their respective quality) is inherently scientifically unsound—but that principle runs completely contrary to the current practices of the media, and scientific institutions and publishers, who usually rush to announce any new single study's results in breathless fashion, without caveats.

epidemiology, with which all investigators and experts in this field have to contend and, which sometimes overwhelm even the best scientists, leading to dietary advice that is widely disseminated and thought to be correct at the time, only to be substantially revised or even retracted, some years later, in light of further evidence.

All of these challenges to nutritional epidemiology mean that there are two important strategies for reducing the chance of wrongly concluding that a food, or pattern of food consumption, is unhealthy or healthy:

1. It is very important to assess the methodological quality of such studies, using the kind of checklists for assessing evidence of causation, which are presented in Appendix 2—or at least look for clear evidence that any structured review of all the relevant studies, used to generate dietary guidelines, has itself done that quality assessment according to widely respected principles (see Appendix 2, 'Useful resources for a critical appraisal tool kit applied to disease prevention'), and then utilized only findings from high-quality studies to come to its overall conclusions.

2. Findings from one analysis, in one cohort, in one setting, require clear replication, ideally in a completely different setting/population, before interpreting them as the basis for global dietary advice about staying healthy.

The examples below have been selected from the recent annals of nutritional science, and widely promulgated dietary guidelines, to illustrate each of the potential pitfalls listed, in interpreting nutritional epidemiology, and laboratory studies of relevance to causation, for generating broad dietary advice for the general population.

Example #1: Measurement error in dietary exposure assessment

It has been known by nutritional researchers for many decades that human memory is an unreliable source of information about precisely what an individual eats. This is not universally important, since some cultures (especially poor, agrarian ones) have so little variation in their diet from day to day and week to week that any recent, well-remembered meal is likely to be nearly identical to all the rest eaten in recent years to decades.[12]

Much epidemiological ingenuity has gone into attempting to reduce this measurement error, in hopes of being able to reduce its adverse scientific effects in cohort studies attempting to link patterns of diet to disease development or death, during long periods of follow-up. However, the two basic data collection tools for the purpose have remained the same for many years. The first is the prospective dietary diary, which is very demanding of study subjects, and generally cannot be relied upon to achieve full and accurate capture of all that is eaten over weeks to months, unless the subjects are unusually motivated. The second major tool to collect dietary data is the mainstay for studies of the general population: the food frequency questionnaire (FFQ). It asks study subjects to report how frequently they have eaten many (100–200) specific foods, over a recent period. This period could be as much as a year or as little as a few days. A seven-day FFQ exploits the inevitably lower recall error for foods eaten only some days earlier, compared to several months earlier. On the other hand, a FFQ asking about foods eaten over the last year is generally accurate for *habitual* eating patterns, which are precisely those most strongly linked to health outcomes. Both methods have well-studied, but rather different patterns of error, which tend to be highest for foods eaten very infrequently, unless they are specifically asked about and happen to be eaten on special holidays (e.g. turkey used to be such a food in North America some decades ago, although now it seems to be eaten year round.) To reduce such measurement error, a FFQ is usually validated and calibrated in each cohort study, for example, against directly recorded food diaries, in a small sample of subjects. Helpfully, epidemiologists have known for many years that the overall effect of such measurement error of exposures in cohort studies, when those exposures are measured with random error (in terms of persons of varying consumption patterns), is *to reduce the likelihood of finding an association*, if one exists, between the exposure (dietary pattern) and the disease outcomes under investigation, in short, such studies are prone to 'false negative' findings, missing evidence of true causal relationships, rather than finding 'false positive' associations that don't actually exist (Rothman et al. 2008).

To accurately estimate the extent of the errors that occur in usual dietary reporting, used for nutritional exposure measurement in epidemiological studies, some investigators have used body measurements (typically in blood) of the precise nutrients of interest after their absorption in the gut, which in some cases accurately reflect the overall recent intake of all foods containing those nutrients. Then these 'absorbed nutrient' exposure data (preferably measured on more than one occasion, over some period of time, in order to capture dietary variation) can be analysed against subsequent disease outcomes, and the results compared to those obtained from analysing self-reported consumption of the foods containing those nutrients, to see how much the errors in the latter exposure data matter to the detection of the diet-disease associations under study. Obviously this works best when the nutrient that can be measured in the body comes only from a specific group of foods easily identified and accurately reported by study subjects, and no other source. A good example is the class of omega-3 fatty acids found largely in oily fish, especially those from cold ocean waters.[13]

In an interesting study comparing these two approaches to measuring body intakes of omega-3s, Mozaffarian et al. (2013) showed that, in contrast to mixed results across *dietary* history studies of oily fish consumption, no doubt related to the errors in such exposure measurements, there was a strongly protective effect (a 27% risk reduction for all causes of death combined) from having high *blood levels* of omega-3s, compared to low levels. This is rather a large health benefit, of a magnitude rarely seen in prevention studies in older persons. It is all the more impressive since all study subjects *were screened to be sure they were not taking any omega-3 supplements. Therefore all observed differences between subjects in blood levels of omega-3s must be largely attributable to higher oily fish consumption and/or the body's conversion of n-3 fatty acids found in flax, canola, soy, and walnuts.* The overall effect observed on deaths from all causes was due almost entirely to an extraordinary 69% reduction in the risk of cardiovascular disease and deaths. Study quality was very high, with over eight years of fastidious, virtually 100% complete follow-up among the 2,692 healthy Americans over age 65 enrolled in the study. Most of the prevented deaths were from coronary heart disease (i.e. 'heart attacks', including those that cause sudden cardiac death by interrupting the electrical cardiac rhythm control mechanism, which omega-3s seem particularly potent at preventing.) Furthermore, the authors point out that these results are completely consistent with RCTs of omega-3 supplements in patients with, or at high risk, of cardiovascular disease, once one corrects for the fact that some such trials were not using a high enough dose of supplements. Furthermore, none of those trials measured baseline omega-3 levels in their subjects' blood, and so those investigators likely provided omega-3s to many subjects who were not in fact in need of them, because they already ate reasonable amounts of oily fish or converted n-3 fatty acids from vegetarian sources to marine n-3s. In the end, while the authors are very temperate and cautious in their conclusions, they convincingly point out that almost no other natural (and rather appetising) dietary option has ever been shown to add so many years of life by and of itself: an average of 2.2 years across all the persons with omega-3 blood levels in the highest fifth of those studied, as compared with the lifespan of subjects whose blood levels were in the lowest fifth.

It would seem reasonable to conclude that, as long as oily fish remain a viable harvest from the sea (e.g. herring is generally considered a long-term sustainable fish) or can be readily farmed (e.g. salmon), they should be on most people's tables a number of times each week. However, the full magnitude of the resultant health benefits was not so clear from studies analysing only what study subjects reported in their food frequency questionnaires— rather, it required a rather expensive set of blood measurements to be done on almost 2,700 persons, who were then followed for nearly a decade for all major illnesses and deaths, before the full benefits of this healthy dietary choice could clearly be seen.

Example #2: Confounding[14] by other characteristics of very unusual eaters

Even in the best-conducted and analysed nutritional cohort studies, such as the acclaimed US Nurses' Health Study directed by top-notch investigators from Harvard University, some findings are regularly published that should be interpreted very cautiously, until clear replication in other high-quality studies is found, ideally in quite different settings and populations. An example is the recent finding (Pan et al. 2013), that the regular consumption of rather large amounts of walnuts was associated with a 24% reduction in the risk of Type 2 diabetes over ten years of follow-up. The authors themselves were very cautious in their interpretation, specifying precisely the concerns that many epidemiologists have had about their finding—described below. However, the popular press and electronic media were not so well informed or cautious, leading to widespread coverage of the study, featuring very confident if not actually exaggerated claims for walnut's health benefits (Hagan 2013; The Telegraph 2013).[15]

To understand why the sophisticated reader might be concerned about such an interpretation of the study, one has to examine in detail the study's large Table 1, on its third page. This table sets out (as all high-quality cohort study publications should) the statistically summarized differences between non-walnut-eaters, and eaters of various amounts of walnuts per week, across more than 30 other dietary patterns and personal characteristics, which might well have influenced these subjects' chances of developing diabetes during follow-up. These characteristics included their family history of diabetes, BMI and reported physical activity levels. Perhaps unsurprisingly, the nurses in the study (only female nurses were included) who ate the largest quantity of walnuts (more than two servings a week) differed on all, but a few of the more than thirty characteristics tabulated, and generally in the same direction: the high-dose walnut-eaters were healthier in almost every way, and especially with respect to their dietary and exercise habits that represent risk factors for chronic diseases such as Type 2 diabetes. Furthermore, only 1,885 nurses out of the total analysed study population of 139,956 ate that highest dose-category of walnuts regularly—less than 2%. Clearly these women were unusual: they had all the characteristics of being very health-conscious, leading one to wonder what other, unmeasured aspects of their lifestyle may have also contributed to their observed lower rate of developing diabetes.

The investigators, fully realising this, did statistically adjust their results for all of these other factors (termed 'potential confounders'). [Statistical adjustment of this kind is the universally accepted approach used in epidemiology to remove from an observed association any confounding, although it is not perfect (Rothman et al. 2008).] This adjustment resulted in a biologically significant decrement in the 39% risk reduction effect observed in the unadjusted data, for the group eating two or more servings of walnuts weekly compared to those eating them 'never or rarely,' to a distinctly less impressive 24% risk reduction attributable 'purely to walnuts' (still statistically significant at the standard p< 0.05 level). As a result, the thoughtful reader of this study is still left wondering:

1. What other features of these very unusual, and presumably self-selected, health-conscious women may not have been measured?

2. Could these unmeasured factors have contributed to what is essentially, after statistical adjustment, a rather modest 24% reduction in diabetes risk? [On the other hand, supporting the case for causation (Chapter 2), the study did find a fairly clear dose-response relationship, i.e. a steady increase in the diabetes-protective effect across the four 'doses' of walnut consumption analysed, ranging from 'never/rarely' through less than one serving a week, to one serving, to two or more.]

The authors do an excellent job, in their discussion, of showing that this observed association also meets other key criteria for causation outlined in Box 3.1, especially 'biological plausibility.' It turns out that walnuts do have a very healthy fats profile in the laboratory, and have been observed in human volunteer studies to improve various aspects of cardiovascular and metabolic function, including some biomarkers linked to the pre-diabetic state and its progression to full-blown diabetes. However, it is unclear whether the free-living and healthy nurses in the study, who report consuming '2 or more servings a week' of walnuts, could be expected to show the same biological effect at that dose, as was seen in volunteer studies typically feeding their subjects much larger amounts of walnuts, under tightly controlled conditions. [One study the authors cite gave diabetics 56 g (two ounces) per day, a dose surely approaching the usual intake of giant squirrels!] The authors also cite an RCT (PREDIMED) of a nut-enriched Mediterranean diet, which showed a reduced risk of both metabolic syndrome (a set of clinical and biochemical imbalances, including blood sugar abnormalities that presage diabetes, which carries a high risk of cardiovascular disease) and Type 2 diabetes, but the subjects in the nut-intervention arm of that study were not just eating a nut-enriched diet, since they were also put on a general Mediterranean diet, the health benefits of which are well established (more on this at the end of this chapter).

In their discussion of other studies on this question, Pan et al. (2013) are unable to point to any other large, high-quality human cohort studies *from other cultures or settings,* implicating walnuts per se as protective from diabetes, presumably because no such analyses have as yet been reported in the literature.[16] Furthermore, we may have to wait quite a while for such scientific replication, since very few nutritional cohort studies internationally have the Nurses' Studies' gigantic sample-size, excellent follow-up for many illnesses (as opposed to merely deaths) and extraordinarily detailed dietary histories (in the Nurses' Study food frequency questionnaires were completed by over 130 000 participants, for over 130 specific foods!) Additionally, Americans, especially those as educated and well paid as nurses, tend to eat a far greater variety of foods than most cultures (as any visit to an American grocery store quickly confirms). It is unlikely that studies done in settings with more restricted traditional cuisines, such as most of Europe, would be able to recruit enough individuals eating such a large quantity of walnuts so as to be able to statistically demonstrate a clear protective effect. Ideally, replication of the Nurses' Health Study finding on walnuts and diabetes should come from a substantially different setting—a society where, and a time-period when, self-selection of persons with healthy lifestyles, affecting many aspects of their health risks, is less likely to have led to confounding by high walnut consumption—for example because walnuts are a significant element in the local traditional cuisine, but not universally eaten in quantity by everyone. [Perhaps a study including a large number of French walnut-oil producers and their employees would be worth mounting!]

However, until there is fully independent confirmation of this benefit of high-dose walnuts, well-trained health scientists and professionals should be wary of the conclusion that we have firm proof from the Nurses' Health Study, and stop short of recommending them to everyone as a diabetic preventive measure. This same caveat should apply to any single study, which shows protective effects from eating an unusual food, especially one, which is widely promoted as healthy (as walnuts have been in the USA for many years)—and therefore likely to be a marker for all sorts of difficult-to-measure health-conscious behaviours.

Example #3: Inadequate laboratory science to show precisely, which nutrients are in which foods, and their health effects

Naturally occurring foods are immensely complex mixtures of thousands of chemical entities, both before and after digestion in our alimentary tracts. Therefore sorting out, which specific nutrients in any given food have precisely which health effects is far from simple, and constantly evolving. An excellent example of this potentially widespread problem is the shifting official dietary guidelines over the last fifty years on fats, and particularly the unfortunately mistaken advice given to millions in the 1950s and 1960s to reduce their consumption of animal fats by substituting margarine for butter. While readers younger than middle-aged will not remember the ubiquitous presence of margarine on dining tables of that era, the older amongst us can readily recall the stunningly bad flavour of the early versions of this ersatz manufactured food. Fortunately for our taste buds margarine is no longer in favour among most nutritionists, unless it is a 'medicated' product (typically including plant stanols) as part of a specific treatment regimen to reduce serum Low-density lipoprotein (LDL) cholesterol levels. That shift in thinking has mostly had to do with the scientific advance that first pointed to trans-fats as a hazard in our diet. Trans-fats are a largely unnatural by-product of hydrogenating edible oils to both make them solid ('spreadable') at room temperature, and also (helpfully for manufacturers' and distributors' profits) increase their shelf-life (US Food and Drug Administration 2015a). Within the last two decades, it has become clear that regular ingestion of trans-fats, which are widely found not only in solid margarines, but also in store-bought baked goods, biscuits, and some fast-foods, substantially increases the risk of coronary heart disease and stroke, by accelerating the process of arteriosclerosis ('hardening of the arteries' Chen et al. 2011). The evidence became so convincing in recent years that a number of jurisdictions—New York City, Denmark, and more recently France and, in 2015, the USA (US Food and Drug Administration 2015b)—have banned the addition of trans-fats completely in all foods for sale, with a predicted reduction in cardiovascular disease and death in the range of 20% (Mozaffarian and Clarke 2009), every year into the future, as a result. It is possible to make margarine-like spreads with very tiny amounts of trans-fats; manufacturers of these products are allowed to claim on the labels that the trans-fat content is 'zero' if they contain less than 0.5g per serving. However, the old 'heart healthy', but in fact *heavily hydrogenated* margarines of yesteryear are no longer recommended by up-to-date nutritionists and other health professionals.

While most educated persons know this, far fewer realize that another mistaken piece of dietary advice, with a similar order-of-magnitude potential for causing harm, affected for decades what are now regarded as two very healthy vegetable oils, specifically olive and peanut oils. Because these oils are mono-unsaturated, they were excluded from the then narrowly-conceptualized list of vegetable oils with cardiovascular protective effects, which at that time were thought to consist only of oils high in polyunsaturates (e.g. rapeseed/canola, sunflower, and safflower oils dominate that market). It was only after some decades of unfavourable recommendations about these mono-unsaturated oils that better science showed them to be at least equally protective for cardiovascular disease as polyunsaturates—and in some cases, notably olive oil, to also have many other healthy constituents. There is a great irony here, in that there are virtually no traditional cuisines in the world based on the common poly-unsaturated oils listed above, purely because those oils cannot be readily extracted from the rather small seeds that contain them, requiring large-scale industrial processes for their extraction. However, there are many traditional cuisines based on olive or peanut oils, and in fact those cultures are *not* associated with high rates of cardiovascular disease, indeed just the opposite. As Michael Pollan, the thoughtful science writer on food puts it in his book '*In Defence of Food*' (Pollan 2008, p.148), a useful very general piece of dietary advice, for staying healthy, is 'Don't eat anything in the grocery store that your great grandmother wouldn't recognize and eat.' Depending on how widely travelled and nutritionally experimental your great grandmother was, poly-unsaturated oils would not pass that test for anyone past middle-age today, simply because those oils were not widely manufactured and used anywhere until well into the twentieth century.

Finally, there are at least two other classes of food, which have been the victim of 'mistaken identity' through their wrongful association with elevated serum (blood) cholesterol levels by nutritional science in the last half-century: eggs, and some shellfish. In the case of eggs, it has taken years of careful nutritional investigation to establish that, while egg yolks do indeed contain the largest concentration of dietary cholesterol of any commonly eaten food, that ingested cholesterol (at least at a dosage of an egg or two per day) does *not*—as the egg producers proudly now proclaim in their ads) contribute meaningfully to a person's blood levels of 'bad' LDL cholesterol (which itself is reliably linked, by many decades of convergent multi-disciplinary research, to the risk of cardiovascular disease and death— Chapter 7) (Mozaffarian and Ludwig, 2015; US Department of Agriculture and US Department of Health and Human Service, 2015). Much more important to one's serum LDL cholesterol level is one's own body's manufacture of cholesterol in the liver (which has a strongly genetic determination in some individuals) as well as one's overall dietary intake of saturated (typically animal-source) fats.

Shellfish were also once wrongly forbidden to all patients with high cholesterol levels, and/or cardiovascular disease, but—at least in the case of molluscs such as mussels, clams, and oysters—have since been largely cleared of any causal role in raising the former, or causing the latter. The issue was apparently the inability of more primitive methods of food-chemistry analysis to differentiate between true cholesterol (which comes from animal sources), and other benign sterols from plants that exist in high concentrations in shellfish, partly due to their bodies concentrating them from algae and the rest of the food-chain beneath them (Vahouny et al. 1981). This is good news for those of us concerned about our cholesterol levels or cardiovascular risk, but who also love shellfish. It might also have been suspected, before the food chemists fixed their analytic methods, by those (including most epidemiologists) who are familiar with the international distribution of coronary artery disease, and of shellfish consumption as a major dietary component. If we look at Europe alone, the regions with very high rates of shellfish consumption are coastal areas, especially on the Mediterranean, where rates of coronary heart disease have long been known to be far lower than in more northerly and interior parts of the continent. Of course, many other features of the 'Mediterranean diet,' besides its extensive use of shellfish, are known to be important in conferring its health benefits (those traditional cuisines also tend to use olive oil in preference to any other oil, and include far larger amounts of fruits and vegetables in the daily diet than other parts of Europe (Boffetta et al. 2010). However, one suspects that eating a lot of shrimp, squid, octopus, mussels, and oysters when possible, could hardly have increased cardiovascular risks very much without that being evident in those regions. Indeed, most shellfish are now widely thought to confer risk reductions for such diseases, through their high concentrations of omega-3s, as noted in the first section of this chapter.

Example 4: multiple hypothesis testing, and the role of the media in research dissemination

The discussion above of the Nurses' Health Study implied, quite correctly, that the very competent investigators who run it have published literally hundreds of journal articles and books documenting apparent associations between dozens of nutrient intake patterns, as well as actual specific nutrient intakes, and the many different diseases that their gigantic study is large enough to be able to examine, with adequate numbers of cases to provide statistical reliability. This is also true of the other large diet and health cohort studies around the world, such as the multi-country 'EPIC' cohort in Europe, which has focused almost entirely on diet and cancers, of all types. This situation is ubiquitous in modern nutritional epidemiology. Even the most cautious and well-trained investigators are strongly incentivized (by both their funders, and also by the competitive culture of research institutions) to publish as many different analysis of their cohort's diet and disease patterns as possible, subject to the rather variable rigors of peer-review— our only protection in science from reading low-quality science in normally high-quality publications.[17]

The central weakness of this system of publication is that there is inevitably over-production of studies that describe diet-disease associations that are spurious, the result of either chance alone, or due to specific weaknesses in study design and analysis, such as those reviewed earlier in this chapter. These 'false-positive' studies are usually identified as such in the long run, through their failure to be independently replicated in completely different cohorts. However, this replication can—as argued above for the omega-3 findings of Mozaffarian et al. (2013)—take many years to occur, simply because only a few studies worldwide have the precise scientific requirements for conclusively addressing the research question to, which one study has provided an 'unusual' answer, requiring independent confirmation.

Clearly, in scientific fields such as nutritional epidemiology, it would generally be better for society as a whole if research institutions, especially not-for-profit and public ones, were to avoid trumpeting the findings to the general media of each single observational study of a given diet-disease association, as soon as they are published. Rather, it would be better for the public to hear, in the first media coverage of any new study, from *independent* researchers in the same field, not associated with the study, regarding their reactions to it, The public deserves to hear from authoritative sources whether the findings of such single studies are suspect for any reason—especially why it may have found a diet-disease relationship, which has not been observed before, and is unlikely to be replicated—suggesting that, perhaps it isn't really there. Sadly, that is not how the research world and the media operate most of the time. The best science reporters typically do check what the investigators' peers are saying about any new study, especially where the findings seem rather unusual. However, the influence of such highly sophisticated science writers is usually restricted by their employment opportunities, typically in only the largest and most established newspapers, and a few high-end television and radio networks for more educated audiences. Much of the media, aided and abetted by over-enthusiastic university and research-institute press officers, and sometimes special interest groups (where it serves their purposes—witness the walnut lobby[17]), just report a simplistic 'bottom line' for each new study about food and health (see Chapter 4). There is no incentive for them to develop an institutional memory that would notice (and comment on) the fact that, for example, another study, completely disagreeing with this new one, was published last month by another group of researchers with equally impressive credentials (see Chapter 3).

Thus it is not surprising that popular culture in most developed countries has come to take much 'official' dietary advice, especially that coming from new research findings, with a proverbial grain of salt. While this may be good for the public in some sense, in that it tends to protect them from overly rapid adoption of dietary advice based on only one study, it also creates a climate of general distrust among the public, regarding the trustworthiness of all 'official' dietary advice emanating from expert scientific advisory bodies. This climate is further reinforced whenever there is a major disagreement among experts about what constitutes a healthy diet, which inevitably occurs from time to time, as with all scientific panels, in every field of research.

Campbell and Campbell (2005), in their book 'The China Study' provide a compelling example of a longstanding 'outsider' view (theirs) of how official dietary guidelines often do not fully reflect current scientific knowledge— or even the agreed-upon science, in the view of most experts. They spend several chapters of the book, painstakingly making the case, as very experienced and highly regarded researchers, that high levels of animal-products (meat and dairy) consumption are the major dietary factor underlying the relatively high rates of many chronic diseases (cardiovascular outcomes, diabetes, and cancers of many—but not all—sites) in developed countries. Their most compelling evidence to back up this assertion is a detailed comparison to rural China, where they led a major study of diet and disease. Currently, many authorities would agree with them, although there is not much solid evidence that small amounts of animal products are harmful to our health (World Cancer Research Fund/American Institute for Cancer Research 2007). However, when the elder Campbell attempted to present this argument, and the now-extensive data that backs it up, to the US national body charged with making and updating dietary guidelines for the general population, he was effectively over-ruled. The panel was unwilling to put its neck out, the Campbell's allege, by recommending such a radical departure from the traditional American diet, largely on the grounds that their recommendations would then be ignored.

Their concern was that the US population would regard such an about-face, compared to several prior decades of Food Rules emphasizing the importance of animal products in a healthy diet, as a clear indication of the unreliable (even mercurial) nature of science.

The Campbells' rebuttal to this arguably cynical view is a simple one: ethically, the public deserve to know what would be the healthiest diet possible, based on the best currently available science, even if most of them decide not to follow that advice—for example, because a lifetime of eating meat and dairy products has made them very fond of these foods. Unfortunately, other scientists on the panel effectively 'vetoed' the dissemination of what was to them 'too radical' a recommendation: to reduce animal product consumption in America across the board. Campbell and Campbell (2005) point out as well, lest any of us be naïve, that powerful commercial forces, in the form of the gigantic American and European meat and dairy sectors, would prove themselves powerful opponents of such advice, which would also have its enemies within the US federal Department of Agriculture, where animal husbandry has long been considered the economic backbone of American farming. Indeed, as Moodie et al. (2013) have clearly demonstrated, 'big-food' industries, as well as 'big alcohol' and 'big tobacco', can generally be expected to act as 'major drivers of non-communicable disease epidemics.'

So, what should you eat and drink?

After a full chapter on why much scientific evidence on diet and disease is intrinsically rather untrustworthy, and prone to frequent change, the reader could be forgiven for not knowing where to turn for guidance on his/her next trip to the grocery store or local restaurant. Again, Michael Pollan, after decades of intelligent and critical reading and writing on this topic, has some helpful advice. He suggests we all develop a taste for those regional/national cuisines around the world, which have been in use for thousands of years, and are associated with generally lower rates of chronic diseases such as heart attacks, strokes, Type 2 diabetes, and the commonest cancers of the developed world (breast, colorectal, and prostate in particular, as they are not primarily smoking-related). There are many possibilities here, and they are already being promoted for treatment in patients with established cardiovascular disease and diabetes—less so for cancer patients, since the evidence is not at all clear that risks of recurrence can be reversed by such diets once one is already afflicted (World Cancer Research Fund/American Institute for Cancer Research 2007). The various Mediterranean cuisines of ancient origin—from coastal Portugal, Spain, France, Italy, and Greece, as well as the Middle East—are all currently considered to have multiple healthy features for preventing chronic disease. Far Eastern cuisines, such as more traditional Chinese, Thai, Japanese, and Korean cooking, are also promising sources of healthy and tasty dishes.

There is one caveat here, however: some of these cuisines have been extensively modified to suit what are perceived as Western tastes, by greatly increasing the content of animal products, fats, sugars (and sometimes salt) when served in restaurants, both within and outside of their regions of origin. Indeed, as some of these cultures have developed large wealthy classes, one of the first dietary preferences exercised (now very visible in both East Asia and South Asia) is increased consumption of meat, and animal fat in various forms, and—depending on local tastes—sugar (especially in the form of sweetened beverages such as sodas.) Thus, one would likely reap health rewards from adopting the largely vegetarian diet of traditional Chinese villages, studied in depth by Campbell and Campbell (2005). However one is unlikely to achieve the same sort of disease-risk reductions from mimicking the high-end, and typically more carnivorous fare enjoyed by warlords and emperors of old, and now prominent in Asian restaurants around the world.

Finally, we have only briefly referred above to the critical role of modern food production/manufacturing/processing and retail industries in creating strong consumer tastes for unhealthy, but profitable foods. A full discussion of this issue is beyond the scope of this book, but we refer the reader to the robust and detailed analysis of the Lancet Non-Communicable Disease (NCD) Action Group (Moodie et al. 2013). They document precise parallels between the strategies of 'big food' industries and 'big tobacco' as well as 'big alcohol' private sector firms, in their use of misleading advertising, and in systematically resisting regulation. This is in spite of the fact that, to quote the Lancet NCD Action Group, 'Public regulation and market intervention are the only evidence-based mechanisms to prevent harm caused by unhealthy commodity industries' (Moodie et al. 2013, abstract, p. 670).

We leave the last word on eating to stay healthy to Michael Pollan:

> Eat [real] food, not too much, and mostly plants (Pollan 2008, p. 1).

Decision support tool

Evidence assessment—2D and E.

Considering the individual, community, or population perspectives—1, 3, and 4.

Considering your personal perspective—1.

Quiz

A 1981 review published in Nature made a strong case that dietary beta-carotene was inversely linked to cancer (particularly of the lung) based on a plethora of epidemiological evidence (Peto et al. 1981). This article was subsequently cited as the motivation for several well-known RCT studies (Omenn et al. 1996; Alpha-Tocopherol Beta Carotene Cancer Prevention Study Group 1994) that gave smokers beta-carotene supplements, hypothesising that it would decrease lung cancer rates. However, the trials were stopped when it became clear that supplementation was actually increasing the incidence of lung cancer in the treatment group. What are some of the potential errors in reasoning that may have occurred in these RCTs, based on what appeared to be sound epidemiological evidence?

Once you have a list of potential reasons why the reasoning may have been erroneous, read this reflective piece (Greenwald 2003), which describes the lessons learnt from these studies to see if you agree.

Preventing chronic diseases by risk factor detection and treatment: what every health care consumer needs to know

Under what conditions can modern medicine reduce the future risk of chronic disease in individuals?

In Chapter 3, a set of criteria was presented to define what constitutes clear evidence of disease causation (Box 3.1). To be considered causally related to a disease outcome, a risk factor has to meet almost all of these epidemiological and non-epidemiological criteria for causation. Otherwise, measuring a suspected risk factor and changing it, especially with individualized medical treatments, would be unethical. The reasoning here is that robust evidence is needed that reducing the risk factor, whether it is stopping smoking, reducing overweight, improving diet, increasing physical activity, reducing serum cholesterol levels, or controlling high blood pressure, will lead on average, to clear health benefits from reduced risks of future disease, as well as acceptable risks and costs. The most important criterion for causation, when recommending a significant preventive intervention, is therefore #8: '*Reversibility—evidence that risk factor modification does reduce disease risk.*' Putting patients with a chronic disease risk factor through a programme of major lifestyle change, let alone a long-term prescription for a cholesterol- or blood-pressure-changing drug every day, for what is usually the rest of their lives, carries a strong ethical requirement with it. That requirement is consistent findings, from high-quality experimental studies, ideally RCTs of net patient benefit from the risk factor treatment. In short, physicians and patients need a measure of certainty that this intervention does indeed reduce the future risk of the disease in question, *by a sufficient amount to be worth the risks and costs involved.*

It is this last issue around which controversy often arises. The arguments for and against medical treatments to modify chronic disease risk factors can become heated when the treatment requires the use of either drugs or major changes in lifestyle, such as extreme diets or intensive physical activity programmes. Such treatments can themselves carry significant risks to health, even though chronic disease risks may in fact be reduced by complying with them.

On the other hand, 'naturalistic' recommendations to the general population for reducing future disease risks (such as 'eat at least five helpings of fruits and vegetables daily', or 'reduce dietary intake of refined salt, carbohydrates, and saturated fats to well below the levels currently consumed in wealthy countries', or 'keep physically active, enough to avoid weight gain in adulthood') are considered by most health experts to carry little or no risk of harm. That is because they represent merely a course-correction in the unhealthy direction in which modern post-industrial life has taken us, back towards the more 'natural' diets and physical activity patterns for which evolution equipped us. Of course the 'natural' nature of such treatments does not necessarily mean that they are effective: one can, and should, question whether compliance with such 'hygienic'[18] advice (as opposed to purely medically prescribed treatments) is merited, given the effort required, attendant personal costs, and potential lost-enjoyment-of-life. Even for such apparently benign lifestyle advice, there is an ethical imperative for health professionals to insist on high-quality evidence that such measures actually do lead to improved health, via reduced disease risks in the future. Otherwise they are guilty of unscientific practice, which eventually affects credibility with the public.

It is generally true that it is safe to adopt traditional dietary, physical activity, and other health-related practices, which have evolved within major cultures over lengthy periods of time, especially cultures which have thrived (for a clear example, see Box 7.1, 'Does a Mediterranean diet prevent cardiovascular disease?'). However, this is not always the case. Some traditional cultures have adopted dietary habits, for example cannibalism among the Fore people of New Guinea, which did harm their health. In that case the health threat arose through the transmission, via eating human brains of a neurological disease, kuru. [Kuru, like bovine spongiform encephalopathy (BSE), the human form of which is variant Creutzfeldt-Jakob disease, is caused by prions, abnormal self-replicating proteins that are not destroyed by normal cooking.] Kuru gradually destroyed the brains of the Fore brain-eaters. While cannibalism could hardly be considered a mainstream dietary habit in human culture, it serves as a warning that some longstanding 'natural' traditions can indeed be harmful. Other, less dramatic examples abound of specific traditional foods, which though tasty and nutritious, contain slow poisons or parasites, typically those which

Box 7.1 Does a Mediterranean diet prevent cardiovascular disease?

In a remarkable example of how to robustly demonstrate the health benefits of a culturally-traditional diet, used for thousands of years by hundreds of millions of persons, Estruch et al. (2013) randomized 7,447 Spaniards at high risk of CVD, age 55 to 80 years and 57% of them female, to either follow:

- A traditional Mediterranean diet, supplemented with a specially prepared and supplied extra-virgin olive oil
- A traditional Mediterranean diet supplemented with mixed nuts.
- A low-intensity dietary advice regimen urging study subjects to reduce their overall dietary fat.

In a statistically exemplary analysis of the primary outcome—the rate of any major cardiovascular disease event (heart attack, stroke, or related death), the authors showed, beyond any shadow of a doubt, that the first group, following the Mediterranean diet with supplemental olive oil, experienced 30% fewer major CVD events, compared with the group eating that same diet but supplemented with walnuts and hazelnuts, and 28% fewer events (not statistically distinguishable from the 30% effect-size just mentioned) compared with the fat-reduced diet group—with no diet-related adverse health effects being reported. The beneficial effects of the olive-oil-supplemented diet were so strong that the trial was stopped for ethical reasons after a median follow-up of only 4.8 years. The remarkable thing about this finding is that the study was executed in Spain, where many people still follow a reasonably traditional Mediterranean diet. This implies that the effects seen would have likely be even larger had the study been done in a setting (such as the UK or North America) where most of the population does not consume such a healthy diet! Furthermore, measures of various biomarkers in the blood of the study subjects showed that there was very good dietary compliance in both the groups randomized to Mediterranean diet and either extra-virgin olive oil (50 g per day more than controls) and nuts (6 servings per week more than controls). So these two treatment diets were clearly palatable. Finally, the clinical efficiency of the olive-oil diet was pretty much similar to that achieved in practice from use of a daily prescribed drug—e.g. statins—to reduce 'bad' cholesterol levels and thus CVD risk: 333 person-years of dietary treatment for each clear beneficiary whose major CVD event was averted, versus 250 person-years of treatment for statins, based on a highly cited summary of 22 statin trials (see Box 7.2).

act over such long periods that traditional people did not make the link between eating them and becoming unwell.[19]

On the other hand, indefinite long-term *drug* treatment, for chronic disease risk factors is rather a different matter. Here, it can readily be appreciated that risks could outweigh benefits. Examples of chronic disease risk factors currently widely treated with daily drugs, usually for many years to decades, include: serum cholesterol levels, high blood pressure, and slightly raised (but not frankly diabetic) blood sugar (glucose) levels. The debate around drug treatments to modify these risk factors centres on the issue of *what **level** of the risk factor should be medically treated, so as to ensure that:*

◆ Benefits outweigh risks, based on long-term follow-up of comparable populations of persons on and not on that treatment. This follow-up must include a full assessment of the benefits, in terms of reducing the risk of the target diseases, as well as any unintended side-effects of the treatment. As has already been discussed, side-effects are rarely fully known for any new drug, vaccine, or other medical intervention until many thousands of persons have been so treated for a number of years, and carefully observed for the occurrence of both risks and benefits.

◆ The net cost per unit of overall improvement in health is reasonable, as measured in standardized units such as 'quality-adjusted life-years (QALYs)'[20] or 'disability-adjusted life-year'. [This cost is borne by different purses in different settings, in terms of its public versus private burden, but the general rule is that the net cost-per-unit-health-benefits, should be widely accepted as worthwhile, and competitive with other routine investments for health improvement, in societies at a similar level of wealth (Appleby et al. 2007)].

Cardiovascular disease prevention in well persons: an unending controversy

A quarter century ago, one of the authors (JF) participated in a structured review of the evidence on cholesterol-lowering treatments, for the province of Ontario, Canada. The review was done to provide guidance to physicians, their patients, as well as the publicly-funded health care system, on what levels of blood cholesterol (both 'good': HDL, and 'bad': LDL) warranted the various specific lifestyle and drug treatments then available. The major monograph from that work is still a good read (Toronto Working Group on Cholesterol Policy et al. 1990). One cannot use the details of that 1990 analysis to decide on the thresholds for modern drugs, e.g. statins, to modify cholesterol levels, because that family of cholesterol-lowering agents has become much more potent, and far less costly. Indeed, that is the reason that statins are now ubiquitously used as first-line agents throughout the world to prevent cardiovascular disease (CVD) in well persons at risk, as well as to improve prognosis in persons with existing CVD, This price reduction has occurred because the older statins are now off-patent, and thus cheaply available as generic agents.

The 1990 report is still informative because it used sound clinical epidemiological reasoning, which subsequently became widely accepted as best practice, to decide what *level* of future cardiovascular disease risk warrants indefinite drug treatment to reduce LDL cholesterol. Indeed, that publication took explicit account of the then-accepted cardiovascular risk factors that a physician could routinely detect in a patient (including age and sex, blood pressure, smoking status, diabetes history, etc.). That approach meant that the report's recommendations were, unlike many expert panels' recommendations at that time, based on clinicians performing a baseline assessment of overall cardiovascular risk in all patients, before initiating risk factor management, including all risk factors pertinent to each patient. The 1990 report also considered risk-benefit analysis, to be sure that benefits of treatment outweighed potential risks. Interestingly, however, the most common risks of statins for cholesterol-lowering were not yet documented at that time, a key point the authors will return to below. The report by the Toronto Working Group on Cholesterol Policy et al. (1990) also performed cost-effectiveness analysis, using basic health economic methods, to assess whether the health benefits of cholesterol treatment, at each level of baseline cardiovascular risk, represented a competitive investment of health care resources for the time.

The key logic in the 1990 cholesterol treatment recommendations is still true today. Cardiovascular risk is strongly related to age, and to being male, until well after women pass through the menopause. Therefore, starting long-term drug treatments to reduce those risks is much less attractive in very young adults, especially women. [Treatment of children was not addressed in that report; it is still a contentious issue, unless the child has clear evidence of a genetically determined syndrome that results in greatly raised 'bad' cholesterol levels (US Preventive Services Task Force 2007)]. Long-term statin treatment, even at today's much-reduced price for the drugs per se, only becomes a competitive investment once patients approach middle-age, unless their cholesterol levels are so out of whack, usually due to an uncommon genetic disorder, that there is a clear and imminent threat to health. Revealingly, the 1990 report by Naylor et al. (Toronto Working Group on Cholesterol Policy et al. 1990). had to contend with three key considerations, in recommending long-term drug treatment for cholesterol to reduce cardiovascular risk, which are still critical today:

◆ The precise benefits of cholesterol-lowering, especially for lengthening life, which can vary across age-groups, women, and minority ethnic and racial groups, all of whom have not been well studied.

◆ The precise risks of taking such drugs for years to decades, and the uncertainties of those risks.

◆ The full costs, to both the patient and any publically funded health care system, of taking powerful prescription drugs such as statins, on a daily basis, usually for many years.

The 1990 analysis was further informed by a fact not always explicitly considered by many subsequent analyses of this sort. As pointed out earlier, some decades are likely to elapse, for anyone starting statins prior to age 40, before any significant benefit would be experienced. This delayed benefit occurs because *cardiovascular disease risk stays very low until after mid-life,* except in rare cases of genetically sky-high risk factor levels throughout life, as already noted. That fact was, and is today, a clear deterrent to starting treatment in younger adult patients with common, garden-variety elevations of 'bad' (LDL) cholesterol—those *not* carrying a specific, but uncommon gene, that causes particularly high cholesterol levels. This basic reasoning behind a more conservative approach to younger patients, and especially women, is unchanged today: well persons not likely to benefit for many years from such preventive treatment must not experience unacceptable risks from that treatment, which are typically experienced in the shorter run.[21]

Current UK NHS and USA practice guidelines for the preventive treatment of risky cholesterol levels are no longer based, as was the case in the early 1990s, on specific cholesterol-level and age/gender cut-offs for initiating intensive treatments such as daily statins. Rather, age, sex, and other key cardiovascular risk factors (e.g. smoking, blood pressure, blood cholesterol levels, diabetes history, and family history of CVD) are now routinely folded into a more sophisticated calculation of each patient's overall CVD risk, through 'CVD risk calculators.' These calculators are freely available online; they utilize over a half-dozen risk factors' values in a given patient, to predict that patient's pre-treatment CVD risk, typically over the next decade.[22] Guidelines then provide CVD risk cut-offs, or thresholds, for starting intensive cholesterol treatments such as statins. As already noted, these thresholds have *shifted downward markedly* in the 25 years since the Toronto Working Group on Cholesterol Policy et al. (1990) report. That shift has occurred because the scientific evidence-base on the benefits, risks, and costs of such treatments, in well adults, has substantially changed:

• Many more high-quality controlled trials of statins, of several newer molecular varieties, have been completed in the intervening 25 years. As a result, the health benefits of this treatment, in terms of the reduction in subsequent risk of heart disease and stroke, as well as overall mortality, have become much more precisely quantified, although there are still unanswered questions about statin effectiveness in subgroups such as women, older adults, and some ethnic and racial minorities. This is simply because we still do not have as many high-quality controlled trials that included large numbers of such persons.

- Arguments in favour of statin use, in patients at lower CVD risk, have been marshalled by expert panel after expert panel, more than a dozen of them internationally since 1990. This is particularly the case in the USA, which has a history of more aggressive prevention guidelines for almost all diseases and interventions (more on this later in Chapter 8, on cancer screening). Consequently, an entire generation of physicians has come to believe, that statins are 'very safe indeed,' although convincing, high-quality evidence in that regard has, remarkably, really only been pulled together in the last few years, and is still contentious (National Institute for Health and Care Excellence 2014; Thompson et al. 2014);

- The retail cost of older statins, which have come off patent protection in the last decade, has dropped precipitously, and now amounts to as little as £16 (US$25) annually for the cheapest generic brands, even for 'high-potency' statins such as atorvastatin, a low dose of which (20 mg daily) can reduce CVD risks by 40%; furthermore, the routine laboratory monitoring of potential muscle, blood, and liver side-effects of statins, repeated indefinitely into the future in all patients on statins, has recently been deemed not cost-effective (National Institute for Health and Care Excellence, 2014), so the indirect costs of 'statin supportive care' have also come down.

As the recommended baseline-risk-thresholds for indefinite drug treatment of cholesterol levels in well persons kept dropping over the last 25 years, it was inevitable that disagreement would eventually surface among medical experts, sooner or later. Predictably, a major controversy has now broken out, as to whether newly proposed CVD risk thresholds, in authoritative, 'evidence-based' guidelines issued in both the USA (2013) and the UK (2014) have gone too far, by recommending that a large fraction (one quarter to one-third) of the currently healthy adult population, from mid-life onwards, should take statins or similar agents every day, indefinitely. The specific concern of the 'guideline sceptics' is that, for the millions of persons in the developed world with CVD risks just above the new treatment threshold, the absolute risk of overt CVD is, first, rather low, and secondly that their first CVD event (heart attack or stroke) is likely to be decades away.

Adding fuel to the fire of the controversy, senior cardiovascular epidemiologists in the UK have argued that:

♦ Statins are entirely safe and effective, in terms of the risk of their side-effects compared with their benefits, in terms of the cardiovascular risks they reduce.

♦ Precise assessment of individuals' future cardiovascular risks is fraught with error, and medically expensive.

♦ Everyone over 60 (perhaps a bit earlier in men, and a bit later in women) should thus take statins daily, without prior assessment of any risk factors, including their blood cholesterol levels (Ebrahim and Casas 2012; Wald et al. 2011; Wald and Morris 2014). Indeed, one major leader of cholesterol-lowering drug trials in the UK has been quoted in the popular press as recommending long-term statins for all Britons over 50 (Hope 2012).

The tipping point in the controversy occurred in the UK in 2014, after the publication in the prior year in the USA, of much more aggressive cholesterol drug-treatment guidelines. The US guidelines were authored by expert panels appointed by the American Heart Association and the American College of Cardiology (Stone et al. 2014). Critical comment promptly ensued in the UK. However, the real storm of British scientific and professional disagreement erupted when the UK's National Institute for Health and Clinical Excellence (NICE) issued a draft set (finalized, in July 2014) of just slightly less aggressive recommendations for treatment of high cholesterol, in terms of who should be put on 'intensive' lifestyle treatment with diet and physical activity, and then, if their LDL cholesterol levels do not come down enough, offered long-term high-potency statin treatment. In both the USA and UK recommendations, the selection of well persons for intensive cholesterol reduction was based on a calculated future risk threshold for developing overt CVD or dying from it, using risk-prediction calculators such as those described.[22] In the UK the threshold for intensive cholesterol-lowering treatment with statins shifted from a 20% chance in the next 10 years to a 10% chance (National Institute for Health and Care Excellence 2014). In the 2013 US guidelines, that threshold was shifted even further: from 20% to 7.5% over the next ten years (Stone et al. 2014). Estimates of the UK population affected by the former change, as recommended by NICE, suggest that the number of British adults eligible for statin treatment under the new draft guidelines will increase by about 5 million well persons (with a total future target population representing about 25% of the adult population age 45–74). [In recent years, only about 7 to 8 million UK residents have actually been taking statins at any one time. Many physicians and patients do not comply with even the current, more conservative guidelines, of which more will be said later (Boseley 2014).]

Objections immediately arose from some highly qualified researchers, many health professionals, and some thoughtful taxpayers [statins are freely available at no cost in the UK to the elderly, those on social assistance, and those with various specific conditions] (Abramson et al. (2013)—*some details of which were later corrected, after an independent tribunal recommended this action, rather than full retraction of the Abramson article—* Godlee 2014a,b); many subsequent letters to the Editors of the BMJ, cited in Godlee (2014a); Goldacre et al. (2014). These vigorous verbal tussles culminated in a tense exchange between eminent physicians and researchers on both sides of this question, in the summer and autumn of 2014 (Armitage et al. 2014; Thompson et al. 2014).

Economic models of this risk-threshold change have indicated that full compliance with the new NICE guidelines would incur a substantial cost to the NHS of £52 million annually (Boseley 2014). The upshot of the criticisms of the new UK guidelines is that they will cause additional millions of adults to start indefinite daily drug treatment, converting them in one stroke of the prescription pen from well people into 'patients,' for the rest of their lives, at significant cost, without commensurate benefits in those at the lower end of the new range of CVD risk targeted for treatment. Specifically, the concern of the guideline critics is that many of those newly targeted by the revised guidelines, especially those at baseline CVD risks between 10 and 15% over the next ten years, are unlikely to experience a clinically important benefit in that time-frame, *because their baseline (pre-treatment) risk of cardiovascular disease is just too low.*

To get a better idea of the implications of typical risks of CVD in the next 10 years, in older adults, the authors need to introduce a simple metric widely used in clinical epidemiology to summarize the full 'effort required to prevent one adverse health event.' That metric is 'the number needed to treat' (NNT). It is calculated from statistical summaries of the results of many high-quality randomized control trials (RCTs)—meta-analyses, covered in Chapter 4. Box 7.2 and Table 7.1 explain its meaning, how it is calculated, and provide specific examples related to CVD prevention.

How do these NNTs compare with those of widely accepted preventive treatments now routinely prescribed by doctors throughout the developed world? As a benchmark in chronic disease prevention, long-term drug treatment for *mild* hypertension (high blood pressure at the level of 140–160 mmHg systolic, over 90–99 mmHg diastolic) has *until recently* been widely accepted, as 'worthwhile' in terms of its NNT (Wright and Musini 2009). That NNT, about 600 person-years of first-line drug treatment to prevent one serious death from any cause related to hypertension (Ogden et al. 2000), is higher than all the NNTs shown in Table 7.1 for statin treatment. However, drug

Box 7.2 The number needed to treat (NNT): a useful summary measure of the clinical efficiency of prevention or treatment to prevent disease

Number-Need-to-Treat (NNT) was first described by Canadian epidemiologists more than 25 years ago (Laupacis et al. 1988). As a worked example of its use, a well-done meta-analysis, by the Cholesterol Treatment Trialists' Collaborators et al. (CTTC 2012), summarized 22 high-quality RCTs of statin treatment, for primary prevention in persons with no prior CVD. By achieving approximately the average reduction in LDL cholesterol levels produced by statins (about 1 mmol per litre of serum—the liquid portion of blood, without cells or clotting proteins), the following reductions occurred, across all these RCTs, in the subsequent incidence of major adverse CVD events (e.g. heart attack, or major cardiac surgery to prevent one; stroke; or death from a cardiovascular cause), leading to the NNTs (see Table 7.1).

Table 7.1 NNTs for statin treatment (by baseline CVD risk)

Primary Prevention Subpopulation, by Baseline Risk of a Major CVD Event over the next 5 years*	Risk of CVD Events per year: Control Group ('C') – No Statins	Risk of CVD Events per year: Statin-Treated Group ('T')	NNT = Reciprocal of difference in Risk = 1/(C-T)
Very low risk (<5%)	0.53%	0.35%	555
Low risk (5 to 10%)	1.53%	1.02%	196
Medium risk (10 to 20%)	2.98%	2.52%	217
High risk (20 to 30%)	5.28%	4.40%	114
Very high risk (> 30%)	8.16%	7.29%	115
All 22 RCTs' primary prevention participants	1.84%	1.44%	250

*Note that this baseline risk of a major CVD illness or fatal event is expressed over the next five years of the patient's life, rather than the next 10 years (the basis for the recommendations summarized in the standard CVD risk calculators, such as the QRISK2 instrument cited later in this chapter). There is no sleight of hand here; the authors of the Lancet meta-analysis had to accommodate the fact that very few of the 22 RCTs they summarized had median durations of follow-up, across their recruited subjects, as long as a decade. Whenever NNT is calculated, it is important to incorporate the period over which the treatment must be taken to prevent one adverse health event—which is the figure calculated in the far-right column: the number of persons who must be treated to prevent one CVD event, for each year of treatment—i.e.

it is the number of persons-years of treatment needed to yield clear beneficiary, whose CVD event was averted.

Source: data from *The Lancet*, Volume 380, Number 9841, Cholesterol Treatment Trialists' Collaborators et al., 'The effects of lowering LDL cholesterol with statin therapy in people at low risk of vascular disease: meta-analysis of individual data from 27 randomized trials' pp. 581–90, Copyright © 2012 Elsevier Ltd, http://www.sciencedirect.com/science/journal/01406736.

To summarize Table 7.1, persons starting statin treatment at the five respective levels of CVD risk shown, experience the NNTs in the far-right column. The NNT is simply the reciprocal of the proportion of each risk-group who will benefit (i.e. have a CVD event averted) during each year of treatment: the number of person-years of treatment per beneficiary. Clearly, that proportion is strongly related to the baseline risk in the first column. The higher the baseline risk, the more efficient the treatment, as reflected in a lower NNT. This simple relationship was recognized even before Naylor et al.'s 1990 report. The relationship is roughly evident in the table, but there is not nearly as much change in NNT between the very high/high risk groups and the low to medium risk groups, as there is in moving to the very low risk group (NNT of 555).

Excellent instructional modules about NNT are available online, from sources such as the Centre for Evidence-Based Medicine at Oxford University: http://www.cebm.net/number-needed-to-treat-nnt/. Readers should be aware, however, that NNT also has its critics (Hutton 2009; Smeeth et al. 1999).

treatment for isolated mild hypertension is now being actively questioned by leading researchers as a worthwhile preventive activity, unless the patient has other risk factors that confer a higher baseline risk of CVD (Diao et al. 2012; Gueyffier and Wright 2014; Martin et al. 2014). This criticism is made all the stronger by the fact that, like only mildly elevated LDL cholesterol levels most mildly hypertensive patients can be successfully treated by diet and physical activity alone, if their motivation can be sustained.

It is noteworthy in Table 7.1 that one has to have a baseline CVD risk above 20% over five years to experience NNTs of about 100 per person-year of statin treatment, which are twice as attractive as the NNTs, of about 200, in the next two lower-risk groups. In other words, there is a natural break-point in the CTTC data in Table 7.1, where the NNT shifts markedly, within the range of moderate CVD risk levels, which are often considered as suitable for statin treatment to achieve primary prevention. (Note that, at least to date, no expert panel in any country is recommending routine statin treatment for the lowest-risk group in the table, with an NNT of 555).

Further statin controversies—side-effects

Contributing to the wave of UK resistance, to the more aggressive draft cholesterol treatment guidelines issued by NICE in 2014, is a set of recent articles in highly-respected medical journals, suggesting an additional legitimate concern (Carter et al. 2013; Culver et al. 2012; Hippisley-Cox and Coupland 2010; Macedo et al. 2014; Mills et al. 2011; Sattar et al. 2010); with contrary evidence also being presented (Cholesterol Treatment Trialists' Collaborators et al. 2012; Kohli and Cannon 2011 Reiner 2013; Ridker et al. 2012—among others). That concern is the strong likelihood that significant major side-effects, such as type 2 diabetes, as well as less dangerous, but potentially activity-limiting symptoms of muscular discomfort, mild cognitive dysfunction, and perhaps erectile dysfunction in men, have not been systematically studied—or at least accurately reported—in the dozens of RCTs of statins currently found in the peer-reviewed literature (Thompson et al. 2014). The particular concern here of those critiquing the NICE guidelines is that the majority of these trials were funded by the pharmaceutical industry, as part of regulators' required documentation of efficacy, and safety, for the drugs' licensure. Detailed examination of all the data collected in these trials, down to the (anonymized) individual-level trial-participants, has been granted to only a limited number of experts in the field; those data are not in the public domain (Godlee 2013, 2014b; Thompson et al. 2014). These trials were well designed and conducted to count the *benefits* of treatment, in terms of reductions in cases of serious cardiovascular illness, and deaths from any cause. However, they were not designed to capture all cases of major illness (even if hospitalized), which occurred in the treatment and control arms of each trial, especially illnesses due to diseases of the body's non-cardiovascular systems—in which many statin effects are now known to occur. Thus, it has been argued by the critics of the new NICE recommendations, the scientific evidence base on which these recommendations were based is potentially biased by its systematic under-reporting of any non-cardiovascular symptoms or full-blown illnesses, which might have been caused by statins (or—one notes—prevented by statins, as has been alleged for dementia after statin use: see below). Further, those critics argue that some such potential side-effects of long-term statins, such as type 2 diabetes, are now solidly established, from more sophisticated recent studies, to occur more often after statin use, and to almost certainly be caused by statins. Box 7.3 provides a detailed analysis of how various sorts of study designs, with varying strengths and weaknesses have been used to address the question of statin side-effects, including diabetes. These studies are a useful worked example of how tricky it can be to obtain solid scientific evidence that a specific exposure, in this case, the taking of statins, *causes* specific effects.

Box 7.3 How do we know that statins (rarely) cause diabetes?

The best current estimates, from the two most sophisticated studies, of overall average extra risk of type 2 diabetes due to statin use are:

◆ *Across the largest assembled set of such side-effect studies, of all study-designs*: 31% more often (Macedo et al. 2014) from studies of all designs (not just RCTs.) This estimate is therefore liable to error, due to uncontrolled confounding—the likelihood that underlying factors differing between statin users and non-users, are driving the observed excess risk; these factors are very hard to control for in observational, non-randomized studies. However, these studies tend to be better designed to capture all new cases of diabetes occurring after statin initiation and during the same time-period in controls, which not all RCTs were designed to do. These higher-quality studies carefully follow up all study subjects for longer periods, both on and not on statins (this can also be done for persons previously enrolled in statin trials—see next paragraph), with full counting of a wider set of disease outcomes, often through record-linkage to routinely collected hospitalisation, prescription, and ambulatory-care data (Macedo et al. 2014).

◆ *Across only RCTs of statins* (Swerdlow et al. 2015): 12% more new-onset diabetes in statins than in controls over the first four years or so of treatment, when most of the diabetic cases are now thought to occur (Dormuth et al. 2014). This proportionate increase in the rate of diabetes (as a side-effect of statins) translates, when one does the math, into a risk of 5.98% in the statin-treated study subjects, versus 5.39% in the placebo-taking controls, for a difference of 0.59% over 4.2 years of follow-up, leading to a 'number needed to harm' (i.e. NNT for each newly diabetic person harmed) of (1/0.0059) = about 170 persons treated for 4.2 years on average, or 714 (4.2 times 170) person-years of treatment with statins for each person suffering diabetes de novo, as a result. Again, controls included in this analysis were randomized to placebo or 'standard care' only, so the risk estimate is more reliable than in the cohort or case-control studies referred to, which are subject to uncontrolled confounding. However, it is well-known that all these statin trials were not assiduously and consistently collecting all new cases of diabetes that occurred in both statin-treated and control subjects. Thus resultant risk estimates may be understating the true diabetes rates in both arms of the summarized trials. However, Swerdlow et al. (2015)

were also able to provide another plank in the evidence base for statins as a cause of type 2 diabetes, in that they showed that a genetic condition linked to this same disease has similar intermediary biological effects to statins (recall that, in Chapter 3, the authors referred to that criterion for causation as 'biological plausibility').

In a nutshell then, studies of diverse epidemiological design have come to reasonable agreement that statins can occasionally cause diabetes. While one new diabetic case in about 700 person-years of statin treatment may appear to be rather low, it is important to note that epidemiology required more than 20 years of widespread statin use to identify and quantify this risk. The corollary is that it would take the discovery of just one more statin side-effect, of similar frequency and severity, to completely cancel out the net benefits of treatment for patients just above the new CVD risk threshold in the UK, who face an NNT of about 350 person-years of treatment for each CVD event averted. [To simplify that math, if a person's baseline CVD risk is 10% over 10 years, then a 30% reduction in that risk gives an NNT of (10 years of treatment per person × (1/(0.10–0.07)) = 333 person-years. This is just half an NNH of 700.]

To be fair to statins, however, the same 2014 meta-analysis (Macedo et al. 2014), of previous studies of all designs, found that statin use was associated—albeit with some risk of bias due to the inclusion of non-randomized studies—with a 26% *reduction* in the risk of dementia and cognitive impairment, perhaps the most feared health problem of later life. So the statin cup may be at least half full.

The relative efficiency (cost-effectiveness) of statin therapy to reduce CVD risks

As stated earlier in this chapter, even if a given preventive intervention is solidly established as conferring more health benefits than risks, decision-makers must still ask a further question: does the cost per unit of net health benefit represent a competitive use of scarce health-care resources, when compared with the cost-effectiveness of other currently feasible investments in prevention for that population. Detailed methodological criteria, for conducting and assessing the quality of cost-effectiveness studies, are beyond the scope of this book; the reader is referred to one of the many texts in this field (Drummond 1997) or the widely available CASP critical appraisal checklist for critiquing cost-effectiveness and similar health-economic studies, the link to which is provide in Appendix 2.

A summary of the way in which such cost-effectiveness calculations are usually done in the case of statin treatments to lower CVD risk, is provided in Box 7.4.

Box 7.4 Typical costs and health benefits included in high-quality cost-effectiveness calculations for statins to reduce CVD risk

Health benefits and risks

◆ Difference between cumulative incidence (sometimes over a fixed period such as ten years, sometimes over the predicted remaining lifetime of the subjects, given their age and CVD risk factors) of major cardiovascular events in: 1) control subjects not on statins, and 2) statin-treated subjects (ideally obtained from high-quality RCTs.) [Note that this is precisely the data extracted from the CTTC meta-analysis of statin RCTs in Box 7.2: it is in fact the reciprocal of the NNT (number needed to treat) shown in the far-right column of that Box).]

◆ Difference between cumulative incidence, over the same period, of major side-effects of statin treatment, such as type 2 diabetes

Both these 'streams over time' of health benefits and risks are then weighted for their relative 'effect on the quality of life,' obtained from various sorts of basic health economic surveys of persons with and without the conditions in question, to yield 'utility' measurements, which can be multiplied by the likely future time spend with each medical condition, in both statin-treated and control groups. The total 'Quality-Adjusted Life-Years' experienced in the control group are then subtracted from those experienced in the statin-treated group, to yield the net health benefits, on average, per person in each treatment group.

Costs of treatment and cost-savings from disease cases averted and caused by treatment

◆ Direct drug costs (now—at the time of writing in late 2014—as low as £16 annually in the UK for the high-potency drug atorvastatin recommended as the universal first-line treatment for well persons with future CVD risks above 10% over the next ten years, at a low starting dose of 20 mg per day recommended by the July 2014 National Institute for Health and Care Excellence (2014).

◆ The costs of medical supervision of statin users—recently estimated in the 2014 NICE report as about £120 in the first year, and about £100 thereafter, for well persons prescribed statins, for as long as they are on them (typically for the rest of their lives).

◆ Cost savings from all cases of serious disease averted and/or caused by the treatment, based on current health system estimates of care-costs, and often simplified to include only hospitalisation costs (although long-term conditions arising from treatment, such as type 2 diabetes, have significant ambulatory care costs over many years, for both the diabetes itself and its common complications, which should be included).

The difference between these summed costs, between the statin-treated and untreated subjects (usually a virtual cohort of men or women with treatment starting at a given age) is then divided into the difference in QALYs experience by the two groups, to obtain the 'incremental cost per extra net QALY gained from treatment (incremental cost-effectiveness ratio: ICER)'. Finally, all these calculations are subjected to 'sensitivity analysis' in which various underlying assumptions are changed to reflect uncertainties in their true value (including the future events' and costs' 'discount rate')[21].

It is a helpful rule of thumb that preventive treatment costs per unit of net health benefits produced (e.g. per QALY) are usually approximately proportionate to the NNT per beneficiary. Since NNTs are, as already noted in Box 7.2, strongly related to baseline risk, it follows that costs per QALY for cholesterol-lowering treatments tend to rise, proportionately to baseline CVD risk—although this relationship is only approximately seen in Table 7.1.

Before summarizing the results of the high-quality cost-effectiveness analysis commissioned by NICE in the preparation of its 2014 Guidance, it is perhaps worth noting that cost-effectiveness analyses of preventive interventions—even those as closely studied epidemiologically, for decades, as long-term statins to reduce the risk of CVD—have historically more often been in disagreement with each other than not. Indeed, it is slightly worrying that NICE's own exhaustive review of all the cost-effectiveness and related health-economic studies of statin therapy for this purpose led to:

◆ The rejection of over *120* published health-economic studies of direct relevance to this controversy, the majority of which were found to have 'serious' or 'very serious' scientific limitations—the rest were outdated or not applicable to the current UK setting (National Institute for Health and Care Excellence 2014, pp. 556–61).

◆ The acceptance, as relevant and of adequate quality to warrant detailed review and commentary in the Guidance, of just *six* health-economic studies, of which five were then re-assessed by NICE-commissioned health economists to have 'potentially serious limitations (National Institute for Health and Care Excellence 2014, pp. 419–29).

One is left with the impression that perhaps those relying in the future on health economic evidence for making such portentous decisions about preventive therapy, affecting millions of persons (in just the UK) for the rest of their lives, should be very cautious about basing their decisions on existing health economic studies. It is small wonder that NICE commissioned its own cost-effectiveness analyses, and then had these independently peer-reviewed as well.

Table 7.2 shows clearly the significant national cost implications, and proportions of the population affected, from bringing down the risk-threshold (shown in the first column) for starting intensive cholesterol-lowering, using drugs such as statins, from 20–10%, and, with even greater implications in terms of risk/benefit ratio and costs, reducing that risk-threshold to 7.5% over ten years (as has been recommended in the USA). Published cost-effectiveness analyses as late as 2011 had concluded that only persons with a baseline CVD risk above about 15% over ten years represented a competitive use of health care resources, based on the usual NHS threshold of less than £20,000 per QALY gained (Greving et al. 2011). However, the July 2014 NICE Guidance includes specially commissioned and very high quality cost-effectiveness analyses that greatly change this picture. Specifically, these new analyses incorporate the greatly reduced costs (since about 2012) of high-potency ('intensity') statins, such as the first-line recommended agent for primary CVD prevention in everyone with a baseline risk over 10% over ten years (atorvastatin 20 mg daily)—currently estimated to cost just over £16 annually for the drug itself.[23] Under this much lower cost assumption, given the expected 40% reduction in CVD risk from daily atorvastatin, even at the relatively low recommended dose of 20 mg as first line treatment, it turns out that (to quote the NICE 2014 Guidance):

> The original (*NICE*) economic analysis found that high-intensity statin treatment using atorvastatin 20 mg (daily) is cost-effective (*i.e. purchases a QALY for less than £20 000*) compared to medium intensity statin treatment for people who do not have CVD (*i.e. for primary prevention*) who have a QRISK score (*ten-year risk of CVD*) above 6.8% . . . At a QRISK2 score of 10% (*risk of CVD over the next ten years*) the ICERs (*Incremental Cost-Effectiveness Ratios*) compared to no treatment were £4,125 per QALY gained for atorvastatin 20mg (*daily*) . . . The base case analysis did not include the potential effects of adverse events other than new-onset diabetes, Two scenario analyses were therefore carried out considering the impact if a greater rate of adverse advents (e.g. muscle pain) in high-intensity treatment causes some people to cease taking statins or to change to a lower intensity. This found that high-intensity treatment (*i.e.*

Table 7.2 Population treatment burdens, costs, and related issues for recent UK and USA authoritative, evidence-based guidance on cholesterol-lowering to reduce CVD risk

Guideline source and threshold to start statins (in terms of 10-year CVD risk of major illness or death)	% Adult population to treat (age range)	Annual statin-related care and drug costs (@ £120 per person) expressed in £ per adult in entire population	Comments
USA: AHA/ACC 2013 (>7.5% 10-year CVD risk)	33% of adults age 40–75	0.33 × £120 p.a. = £40 p.a. per adult age 40–75 in entire population	Many persons at relatively low CVD risk (<10% in 10 years) are much less likely to benefit in a clinically significant way from long-term statins, but could suffer side-effects; costly overall;
UK: NICE 2006–8 (>20% 10-year CVD risk)	8.7% of adults age 35–74 (11% of men and 6.3% of women)	0.087 × £120 p.a. = £10.44 per adult age 35–74 in entire population	Omits to treat moderate-risk (10–20% in 10 years) patients with very attractive cost per QALY of benefits; saves on overall costs;
UK: NICE 2014 (>10% 10-year CVD risk)	25% of adults age 35–74 (30.9% of men and 19.4% of women)	0.25 × £120 p.a. = £30 p.a. per adult age 35–74 in entire population	Intermediate strategy (between those above) in terms of both overall costs and cost-effectiveness; may triple the proportion of population age 35–74 offered statins

with atorvastatin) would still be cost-effective compared to medium-intensity treatment in that situation . . . high-intensity statins (*in particular, atorvastatin*) are the most clinically effective option for the primary prevention of CVD and are cost-effective compared to all other options and so should be recommended (National Institute for Health and Care Excellence 2014, p. 192) (*italics added for clarity*).

In practical terms, this means that the 2014 NICE Guidance has demonstrated that treating everyone with a baseline CVD risk over 10%, with atorvastatin 20 mg daily, represents a very competitive use of UK health care resources at £4,125 per QALY gained—well below the usually accepted threshold of £20,000 per QALY gained. What it means in lay terms is that in the UK, virtually all healthy citizens over 55 are to be offered statin treatment indefinitely, because their cardiovascular risk lies above 10% over the next ten years (Capewell 2014). Overall, the guidance (if fully implemented, which remains to be seen) will lead to 30.9% of 'well' British men and 19.4% of women, age 35 to 74 years of age being offered statin therapy for the rest of their lives—a sea-change in preventive care that will see a massive increase in the proportion of healthy persons prescribed daily statins indefinitely, compared with the NICE 2006–8 guidance (Collins and Altman 2012, Table 5, p. 9).

However, as many authoritative writers have pointed out recently, just because a treatment is technically cost-effective, in terms of being a competitive use of health care resources, does not necessarily mean that it is the most prudent use of those resources, nor the most acceptable policy to key stakeholders. At the end of this chapter, we shall see from those writings that other considerations can and should sometimes trump narrowly technocratic considerations of cost-effectiveness: public/patient and health care provider values and preferences, in this case with regard to indefinite, daily prescription drug use for the relatively low absolute probabilities of benefit implied by the high NNTs in Table 7.1. This is especially the case in the publicly funded—and currently rather cash-strapped—NHS in the UK. Some critics of the new aggressive statin guidance from NICE have in fact suggested that a hidden opportunity cost of this expenditure will be that fewer resources are available to tackle upstream prevention of cardiovascular disease, though policy- and programme-led changes to the incentives around stopping smoking, healthy eating, and physical activity (as discussed in Chapter 5, about the obesity pandemic) (see all Box 7.5).

Box 7.5 Other considerations

Additional doubts on the part of those critical of the NICE 2014 draft guidelines on cholesterol drug treatment have included:

◆ Substantial uncertainty as to *whether persons over 70 to 75 years of age benefit* significantly from taking statins, especially in terms of added longevity (Lloyd et al. 2013). The specific concern is about the quality of life during the additional years, considering that most clinicians would consider 'sudden cardiac death' preferable to cancer or dementia.

◆ There is currently less compelling evidence concerning the *net benefit-risk tally of long-term statin therapy for women and minorities*, especially for improved longevity (National Institute for Health and Care Excellence 2014). This is a result of the fact that drug trials have historically tended to only include white males. Newer studies have included substantial numbers of women (a requirement to be funded by many he major international research agencies, including NIH in the USA) so more data will undoubtedly be forthcoming.

◆ A question which dogs most projections of potential health benefits, from taking statins indefinitely, is the well-documented tendency for ordinary patients to *stop taking pills daily* for conditions such as elevated cholesterol levels that have no current symptoms. This is much less likely to be the case for the sort of persons deliberately recruited to RCTs, who are selected on the basis of likelihood of compliance, so that they are 'good study subjects'. One study of patients over 65 in general practice found that only 25% of well patients prescribed statins, for primary prevention, were still taking the drug after two years (Maningat et al. 2013).[24]

◆ There are significant inconsistencies in the reported rates of various potential side-effects, across published statin trials (Thompson et al. 2014). The overall pattern suggests that (drug) industry sponsored trials may not have ascertained as fully and reliably such symptoms and diagnosed diseases, across their two trial arms, in a comparable fashion.

◆ At least one recent survey of UK GPs found that 57% did not support the new guidelines, 25% did support them, with the rest being undecided (Thompson et al. 2014). Moreover, the GP Committee, which negotiates with the UK NHS for GPs, have formally opposed the 2014 NICE guidelines for statins, until 'this is supported by evidence from complete public disclosure of all clinical trials' data.'

Overall conclusions

Because hundreds if not thousands of pages of scientific papers, journal editorials, commentaries, media stories, and blogs have been written about the statin controversy in just the last few years, it would be unfair to both sides of the argument to attempt to synopsize all the relevant evidence in an authoritative way, in the limited space available here. Such a summary would also quickly become outdated, as new evidence on this issue is being published at a frenetic rate. However, the following, general conclusions about the detection and management of chronic disease risk factors can be made. These recommended 'best practices' apply to the long-term treatment of any medically identified risk factors for subsequent disease, which are themselves not causing symptoms and, which therefore require a high standard of scientific evidence before inherently artificial means of modifying those risk factors are prescribed to large segments of the well population, on a long-term basis, at significant cost.

Given the well-documented tendency for commercially sponsored controlled trials, of treatments that will be sold for profit, to understate the risks and overstate the benefits of such treatments, full and transparent examination of the individual-participant-level data from all pertinent trials should be scrutinized by an independent panel of experts; that examination should establish best-available estimates of quantified risks and benefits of the proposed risk factor modification, under realistic population conditions of use, over realistic time-frames; these estimates should ideally include any credible estimations—to the extent that this is scientifically possible—of differential risks and benefits for particular segments of the population, by age, gender, race/ethnicity, socioeconomic status, or disability/co-existing disease status.

Full disclosure of all scientific uncertainties in that risk-benefit assessment should be an integral part of the assessment, including any doubts of the expert panel about the quality, accuracy, and completeness of the trial evidence available to it, in its deliberation; this standard of reporting is rapidly becoming the norm.

Special measures should be taken to screen *all* prospective members of such expert panels for potential conflicts of interest, which should include receipt of funds, gifts, or other benefits received from parties standing to gain or lose—financially or in terms of influence and reputation—from influencing the content of the panel's final recommendations. Indeed, there is legal research that argues convincingly that mere disclosure of such potential conflicts of interest can be counter-productive, and that it is preferable to simply not allow participation in such decision-making of persons who are clearly potentially conflicted (Bekelman et al. 2003; Cain et al. 2005; Godlee 2013, 2014b; Roseman et al. 2012; Smith 2006; Thompson et al. 2014).

Perhaps the final word on this issue should go to the eminent media columnist and epidemiologist Dr Ben Goldacre. Dr Goldacre has pointed out in a letter to the BMJ in June 2014, concerning the 'statin wars,' that the real need—as described—is for high-quality, transparently-derived data on the benefits, risks, and costs (to various parties, including the state and the patient) of the treatment options, at each level of baseline CVD risk, and capable of being tailored to individual patients *and their personal values and preferences*:

> 'In reality, all patients are different, and—as doctors or as patients—weigh up different factors differently. Some want longevity at any cost; some think that taking a pill every day is an affront to their independence. Some think that aching muscles are a trivial niggle; some think that side effects—even when mild, well-documented, and carefully discussed—are proof that their doctor is a reckless idiot.
>
> When we offer statins, or any preventive treatment, we are practising a new kind of medicine, very different to the doctor treating a head injury in A&E. We are less like doctors, and more like a life insurance sales team: offering occasional benefits, many years from now, in exchange for small ongoing costs. Patients differ in what they want to pay now, in side effects or inconvenience, and how much they care about abstract future benefits. Crucially, the benefits and disadvantages are so closely balanced that these individual differences really matter Goldacre (2014).

Text extract reproduced from Ben Goldacre, 'Adverse effects of statins', *British Medical Journal*, Volume 348, G3306, Copyright © 2014 British Medical Journal Publishing Group, with permission from BMJ Publishing Group Ltd.

Decision support tool

Evidence assessment—2D and E.
Considering the individual, community or population perspectives—1, 2, 3, and 4.
Considering your personal perspective—1.

Quiz

In a new analysis of a small subsample of subjects in the Spanish 'PREDIMED' trial of the Mediterranean (Med) diet plus extra-virgin olive oil, or nuts versus controls (Box 7.1), investigators (Valls-Pedret et al. 2015) reported the following rates for the outcome 'mild cognitive impairment' (MCI) on sophisticated psychometric testing:

Proportion of Trial-Arm Subjects Developing New Cases of MCI (at an average follow-up of 4.1 years after randomization):

Group 1: Olive oil and Med diet: 13.4%.

Group 2: Nuts and Med diet: 7.1%.

Group 3: Controls: 12.6%.

If the numbers of such cases were sufficient to demonstrate statistically significant differences across these cumulative incidence rates of MCI (in this case they were not—the study was too small), then one could calculate, for example, the NNT to prevent one case of MCI by changing to a Med diet with extra nuts.

Question 1: What is that NNT, across the entire period of follow-up reported here?

Question 2: What is the NNT expressed in the more informative format of 'number of person-years of treatment required for the prevention of one MCI case?

Chapter 8

Detecting disease before symptoms begin: the blemished promise of cancer screening

Preamble

Here, again, is the essence of the prostate cancer screening story (Box 8.1).

The authors pointed out in Chapter 2 that some national cultures—notably that of the USA—have a strongly held view that 'more check-ups and testing for well persons can only be a good thing'. The underlying rationale here is the obvious one—any disease that is detected early will have better outcomes. It is tempting to believe this is true for diseases that we all fear, such as cancer. Ironically it is cancers that are particularly likely to fail to meet modern epidemiological criteria for establishing that a screening programme does more good than harm. In this chapter, these criteria are explored to better understand why this is so.

What is screening?

Raffle and Gray (2007, p. 37), in their superb text on screening define it thus:

> Screening is the "testing of people who either do not have (or do not recognize) the [clinical] signs or symptoms of the condition being tested for. In other words, they believe themselves to be well in relation to the disease that the screening relates to". "The stated or implied purpose is to reduce the risk for that individual of future ill health in relation to the condition being tested for, or to give information about risk that is deemed valuable for that individual, even though risk cannot be altered".

Box 8.1 Prostate cancer screening story

The PSA (Prostate Specific Antigen) blood test to detect early-stage prostate cancer has been used in over 75% of completely healthy American men over 50, in the three decades since the 1980s, to detect early-stage prostate cancer. In a conclusive European trial over 180,000 male subjects were followed for over a decade after being randomized to either repeatedly have the screening test or not, the use of this test was finally shown in 2009 and 2012, to lead to a cancer diagnosis for between 33 and 48 *extra* men per one man whose life was actually extended by PSA screening. Most of those 33 to 48 individuals were treated with invasive surgery, radiation or chemo/hormonal therapy, all of which have disabling side-effects. Trial subjects who were clear beneficiaries of testing—i.e. whose death from prostate cancer was prevented by early detection and treatment— numbered (at the latest follow-up) only 1 in about 1,000 men screened every four years, about twice (Barry 2009; Chou et al. 2011; Schröder et al. 2009). Largely in response to this trial, the USPSTF recommended against routine PSA screening (US Preventive Services Task Force 2012b).

Why screening often appears effective when it is not—a personal perspective

One of the authors (JF) contributed a number of articles to the peer-reviewed literature on this topic in the 1980s—all of them critical of under-evaluated screening for various types of cancer (Frank 1985a,b,c; Frank and Mai 1985; Westlake and Frank 1987).[25] For a half-century, many other epidemiologists have also produced scholarly papers on how to critically assess claims of effectiveness and efficiency for screening programmes. However, during this same period, screening programme after screening programme has been introduced, especially in North America, and widely taken up by doctors and patients, with little solid evidence of net benefits (over harms), at reasonable cost. In fact, it is only in the last half-decade that robust evaluations of cancer screening programmes have demonstrated that a test to detect cancers early can actually do more harm than good. While occasional scientific articles suggested this possibility for mammography in women under 50 (US Preventive Services Task Force 2009b), the multi-country European Randomized Study of Screening for Prostate Cancer (ERSPC), published in 2009 (Schröder et al. 2009), was the first high-quality study to demonstrate clearly that a 'simple blood test' for early cancer—Prostate Specific Antigen (PSA)—had almost certainly done harm to more patients than it helped.

Predictably, the reaction to that publication, and a subsequent paper confirming these findings, after an additional few years of follow-up (Schröder et al. 2012), has been mixed. Indeed, considerable resistance to the 'bad news about PSA testing' has continued, particularly in the USA. And the resistance persists even after these and other new studies' results were thoroughly quality-checked digested and expertly summarized as clear practice guidelines. The guidelines were issued by the prestigious, entirely neutral US Preventive Services Task Force who advised against routine screening by PSA for men of any age (Chou et al. 2011; Moyer and US Preventive Services Task Force 2012). In direct opposition to that authoritative recommendation, as recently as early 2014 the US National Comprehensive Cancer Network (NCCN) published updated guidance stating that routine PSA testing of all healthy men should begin at age 45 and end at age 70 (National Comprehensive Cancer Network 2014).

What are the key elements of scientific and professional disagreement around PSA screening, an apparently simple and rather inexpensive blood test? Several counter-intuitive features of cancer screening are relevant here, for they tend to make any screening test for cancer seemingly effective, even if it is not. This is to say, the screening test's benefits tend to look effective with respect to lives apparently saved from the cancer being screened for, and any risks from that testing tend to be undercounted, whether they are from the screening per se (e.g. radiation exposure in mammography) or from the investigation and treatment of screened-positive cases. These *paradoxes* of cancer screening can be more fully described as follows (Raffle and Gray 2007):

◆ Cancer is a disease of great variability from patient to patient, and a key element of that variability is its aggressiveness, which is related to both its rate of growth, as well as its tendency to spread widely in the body (metastasize). Screening tests preferentially detect slow-growing cases of any type of cancer, because those cases remain in the pre-clinical stage, causing no signs or symptoms, for longer periods than fast-growing tumours. Thus one cannot compare cancer cases detected by screening to those that are naturally diagnosed by physicians during their investigation of symptoms in persons who are unwell. Screening-detected cases will always have a better prognosis, even if the screening test is useless (i.e. does not actually reduce mortality or improve quality of life for those screened). Epidemiologists call this *'length (-time) bias'*.

◆ Screening—especially for cancers in older people—often detects very slow-growing and early-stage tumours that would never cause symptoms or disability, let alone death, simply because they would require decades to do so. The person is destined to die of another cause before that time has elapsed. [This is especially true for prostate cancer. Cancer in the prostate can be detected on autopsy of the vast majority of the oldest elderly men, even those who have died of a completely different disease and never had a diagnosis of prostate cancer.] 'Indolent' cases of slow-growing cancers tend to make any set of screen-detected cases do much better, prognostically, even without treatment, because they are so benign. Epidemiologists call this 'over-diagnosis (bias)'. When completely benign cases, detected by screening, are then subsequently medically treated, epidemiologists call that 'over-treatment'. Over-treatment of cancer resulting from PSA testing can be a major problem, as discussed below.

♦ Any set of screen-detected cases has a survival rate, typically measured at one, two, or five years after diagnosis, which is automatically higher than naturally diagnosed cases. This holds true even if tumour aggressiveness is identical in the two case series (screen-detected and naturally occurring cancers) and the screening test is worthless (i.e. does not extend life or reduce future illness). This false appearance of benefit occurs because screening *moves the time of diagnosis,* the start-time of the 'stop-watch' of survival—forward, in terms of the patient's age at, which it occurs. Thus comparisons of 'per cent surviving' at any time-point after diagnosis are not valid, if one is comparing screen-detected and naturally occurring cases; such comparisons will always favour screen-detected patients' survival times, because they are not calculated in a way comparable with that used for naturally occurring cases. Epidemiologists call this 'lead-time bias'.

♦ Comparisons between persons who seek out and comply with screening tests, and persons who self-select not to be screened, are also not legitimate comparisons; such comparisons ignore the well-known fact that persons seeking out preventive care are much more health-conscious in general, and tend to live longer and/or experience less illness and disability than persons not seeking preventive care. Epidemiologists call this 'volunteer (or healthy screenee) bias'.

♦ Finally, there is a particularly vexing social phenomenon for science-based policy-making in screening, termed the 'popularity paradox' by Raffle and Gray (2007, p. 68): *the less accurate the screening test, in terms of both frank false-positive errors as well as its tendency to over-diagnose, the more patients who have undergone it come to believe they have been 'saved from late-stage cancer and death' by screening.* These 'false beneficiaries' of screening then tend to join cancer advocacy organisations (which have historically tended to promote poorly validated cancer screening, even when there was no evidence of net benefit) mistakenly believing that others should be screened as well.[26]

The upshot of these paradoxical features of cancer screening in general is that experts now rely on randomized control trials (RCTs) to provide an 'unbiased'—i.e. valid—statistical estimate of the benefits of screening. Other sorts of study designs, including cohort, case-control, and quasi-experimental studies (see Chapter 5) can legitimately be used to learn about specific aspects of implementing screening programmes in a given jurisdiction, such as: the proportion of the target population actually screened, their compliance after screening with recommended diagnostic tests and treatments for disease cases found, the costs of these outcomes, and to some degree, the side-effects of being screened). However, epidemiologists have come to distrust any evaluation of screening's benefits and harms that is not based on an RCT (US Preventive Services Task Force 2015).

Principles of effective and efficient screening programmes to detect asymptomatic disease (especially cancers)

There are widely accepted requirements for scientifically demonstrating the effectiveness and efficiency of any screening programme. However, in the early days of enthusiastic promotion of new screening tests, these requirements have historically tended to be overlooked.[27] Those pre-conditions for screening programme effectiveness and efficiency have been rephrased by many authors since Wilson and Jungner (1968) first described them in a landmark WHO publication more than forty-five years ago. The essential criteria are updated here and each is presented with a current example of a proposed screening programme, which has failed to meet that criterion:

Common occurrence of disease or condition

The disease or condition to be detected by screening must be common enough, *in the population to be tested,* and its health and economic consequences severe enough, that a reasonably effective screening programme has a chance to achieve competitive 'costs per QALY' (or similar measure of cost-effectiveness—see Chapter 7); cost-effectiveness must include costs of the screening tests, confirmatory diagnostic testing, and related treatments of the 'extra' disease cases detected by screening.

> *Example*: some extremely rare, but treatable congenital conditions would meet this criterion for inclusion in the battery of neonatal screening tests currently done on virtually all new-borns in developed countries, if only they were more common. The cost of the neonatal 'heel-prick' blood test for such very rare conditions must be nearly nothing to make the test worth using in all

new-borns. Thankfully, newer tests are approaching that low level of cost (NHS Screening Programmes 2015).

Pre-clinical phase

The disease or condition to be detected must have a pre-clinical phase when it can be detected before signs and symptoms would typically reveal its presence.

> *Example*: cardiovascular disease experts know that a large fraction of persons suffering their first heart attack, have had no prior symptoms of their underlying coronary heart disease (CHD). Indeed, many patients suffer 'sudden cardiac death' during that first heart attack. Efforts thus far to identify such patients in advance, by screening tests for their pre-clinical CHD have failed, partly because the standard cardiovascular risk factors (discussed in Chapter 7) are not present in a substantial proportion of such cases, beforehand, and partly because sub-clinical signs of narrowed coronary arteries are so common in older well persons, when they are looked for by expensive and somewhat risky imaging such as angiography, that it is not currently sensible or cost-effective to screen asymptomatic persons by directly imaging their arteries (US Preventive Services Task Force 2015).

Improving health outcomes

Any screening programme aiming to actually improve health outcomes must be offered, without major financial or other barriers to patient uptake, together with a *proven-effective and widely agreed-upon treatment* for those testing positive, after confirmatory diagnostic evaluation demonstrates clinically significant disease; furthermore, that treatment must be more effective at the earlier stage of disease detected by screening, than it is at the typically later stage at which patients usually present to care spontaneously (in the absence of screening).

> *Example*: lung cancer screening, whether by x-rays, sputum testing for abnormal cells, or other means, has repeatedly failed to meet this criterion, largely because there were not very effective treatments available for most forms of this cancer until recently, even at the earlier stages potentially detectable by screening. It is also true that this cancer usually stays silent for a long time, and tends to metastasize to the centre of the lung or other organs rather early, making it very hard to improve the prognosis by current methods of screening (US Preventive Services Task Force 2013b).

Screening test acceptability

The screening test itself must be reasonably benign, and acceptable to well persons (in terms of its discomfort, risks, and costs).

Example: in some cultural settings, screening tests involving considerable discomfort have been successfully used, apparently because the disease being tested for is common, and very much feared in that setting; the Chinese practice of having older well persons, even those not at especially high risk of stomach cancer, swallow an inflatable balloon (which is then removed when partially inflated in order to sample the cells of the stomach and oesophagus) probably would not be widely accepted in Europe or North America (where the disease is much less common, and its incidence has been spontaneously decreasing steadily for decades, for reasons not entirely understood) (Liu et al. 1994). A more subtle example is the historically widely promoted practice of breast self-examination in well women, to detect early breast cancer: one of the authors (JF) showed in a short paper in the Lancet, thirty years ago, that this screening test was most unlikely to do more good than harm in women under 35 to 40 years of age. This was because the incidence rate for clinically important cancer in that age group is so much lower than the rates of occurrence of benign tumours of the breast, which do not benefit from early detection, and the full investigation of which (usually by surgical biopsy) is both inherently risky and costly (Frank and Mai 1985). Yet the cultural attractiveness of breast self-examination, once naively thought of as a means of helping women 'control their own health,' meant that this practice continued to be widely promoted until quite recently, when conclusive large trials failed to show any net benefit (US Preventive Services Task Force 2009b)

Natural history of the condition

The natural history of the condition being tested for should be adequately understood, and especially the quantitative dynamics of early-stage cases transitioning to full-blown clinical diseases causing ill health, over the long time-frames frequently involved in screening, and the subsequent treatment of the cases detected by screening.

> *Example*: Cervical cancer screening, historically by Pap smear testing in primary care, has turned out to carry with it a surprisingly high rate of over-diagnosis and over-treatment, of very early-stage cases unlikely to ever cause clinically important disease; a significant proportion of such cases, detected by Pap smears, are thought to resolve on their own, perhaps via elimination by the body's natural defence system. As a result, over-diagnosis is a significant challenge for Pap smear programmes (US Preventive Services Task Force 2012a). Better testing methods, involving, for example, detection of Human Papillomavirus (HPV) infection, which is now established as the underlying infectious cause of cervical cancer, are under active development, partly for this reason.

There is consensus among screening experts that these criteria for effective and efficient screening programmes are as important today as they were when first promulgated by Wilson and Jungner (1968) nearly a half-century ago.

However, the reality is rather different: all new medical technology, as pointed out in Chapter 2, is potentially subject to premature adoption, leading in some cases to iatrogenesis (doctor-caused ill health). Entire health care systems often begin to use new drugs, vaccines, tests, and procedures before we fully know their benefits, risks, and related costs. Where immediate patient benefit is clearly likely, because the patient is very unwell and previously available treatments have failed or are contraindicated, one can more readily accept relative ignorance on the part of medical science regarding technological innovations. However, in the case of screening for early, hidden disease in well persons, no such compelling argument exists. Initiating a new screening programme, especially one targeted at a large proportion of the healthy population, need never be a rushed decision. There is always time to obtain high-quality evidence of benefits, risks, and costs, and consider them carefully, before screening policy is made, and certainly before actual implementation of screening programmes. The authors now turn to what such evidence looks like.

Anatomy of a high-quality screening RCT: dissecting the ERSPC trial

Because of its landmark status, it is worthwhile understanding the precise strengths (and a few weaknesses) of the first RCT of cancer screening to fully document the harms, as well as the benefits of screening: the ERSPC trial of PSA testing for prostate cancer first published in 2009, and updated with an additional few years of follow-up data in 2012 (Schröder et al. 2009; Schröder et al. 2012).

The 'Critical Appraisal' criteria for assessing the quality of any RCT of screening have been provided in Appendix 2, 'Useful resources for a critical appraisal tool kit applied to disease prevention'. They include the standard criteria used to assess the quality of any RCT, as well as a few extra criteria, devised by the authors on the basis of arguments by Raffle and Gray (2007), which are specific to screening trials. In the overview below, key features of the study's design and analysis are summarized to demonstrate just why the ERSPC study is such a high-quality cancer screening trial:

Strength of the randomized study design

The strength of the randomized study design is clearly demonstrated by data presented in the published paper. The paper carefully documents the characteristics of the two groups, randomized to be either PSA-tested regularly (every four years, for a total of just over two tests per subject on average, across the seven participating European countries) or not screened. In the unscreened control group, the policy was simply to treat all prostate cancers, as they naturally presented, according to then-current practice guidelines. The reporting on the comparability of the two groups, in the 2009 ESPRC paper, clearly reveals (Table 1, p. 1324) that the randomization was successful, across 162,243 subjects in the main age-groups of interest: 55 to 69 years at trial recruitment. The comparison shows that randomization successfully produced virtually exactly the same average and median ages in the two groups. Furthermore, the text of the paper shows (p. 1321) that the rates of death from causes *not* related to prostate cancer were identical in the two groups. [Similar death rates would be expected when the intervention is 100% specific to prostate cancer, as is the case with PSA testing (other health risks remain unaltered).] This strong evidence of comparability of the two randomized groups ('arms' of the trial) is important, as is the enormous size of the two arms. Indeed, the ERSPC Trial is one of the largest screening trials ever reported—see below for why this was necessary. The comparability and size reassures us that randomization also achieved precise balance across the two groups for any other factors that might have influenced subsequently observed differences between the groups in the trial's primary outcome—prostate cancer mortality.

Primary outcome

The primary outcome (prostate cancer mortality) was objectively and identically counted in all study subjects. One of the cleverest design features of the ERSPC trial is that all of the seven participating countries have for some decades had well-established cancer registries for their entire population. The trial's subjects could thus be followed at arm's length, and any occurrences of prostate cancer, as well as deaths from it, could be independently counted in a high-quality, objective way, even if some subjects were 'lost to follow-up' in terms of actual contact with study staff. A degree of loss of contact is inevitable in large trials of this size, for example when a subject moves residence without telling study staff. However, great efforts were made in this study to find any such subjects, especially if they moved outside the seven countries, and so escaped surveillance by the cancer registries. In fact, detailed information is provided in the 2009 paper about the precise level of follow-up achieved in both arms of the trial (Figure 1, p.1321 and Table 1, p. 1324, Schröder et al. 2009): practically identical mean and median follow-up times, of 8.8 years and 9.0 years respectively, were achieved in the two groups. This reassures the reader that no special effort, to find lost subjects and ascertain their outcome status, was made in one randomized group, more often than in the other. As well, an independent Data Safety and Monitoring Committee of experts carefully oversaw all aspects of data collection and outcome adjudication (in cases of doubt about the cause of death). That is, they refereed any dubious deaths fairly, as to their cause. Finally, it is virtually impossible to 'blind' subjects in a screening trial to whether they were randomized to receive screening or not. That is because the process of screening itself, and the often invasive confirmatory testing of persons screened as positive, is ethically and practically impossible to hide from the patients undergoing it. Therefore it is important that the primary outcome in such a trial is unlikely to be affected by the placebo effect—in this case, the knowledge that one is being given a preventive intervention. Independently counted cases and adjudicated deaths from prostate cancer, as is normal within well-developed cancer registries, are above reproach in that regard.

Study size

The study was deliberately planned to be large enough, with enough follow-up duration, to find any difference between the two groups in the primary outcome that could be considered of clinical importance was not due to chance alone. This statistical aspect of the study is more technically complex to explain; the bottom line is that the study's protocol, published many years before any results were available, clearly justified the very large sample-size (number of subjects, in each arm) to be randomized. The study's aim was to have a high probability (86%—the 'statistical power' of the study, well above the usual 80%, which is typical in such trials) to find a statistically significant ($p < 0.05$) difference in prostate cancer mortality, between the two arms, of at least 25% of the control arm's prostate cancer mortality rate (a widely accepted standard for a minimum effect of interest, in terms of cancer mortality reduction, achieved through screening.) In the end, although the study was planned to require follow-up until 2008, it was stopped two years early, because sequential statistical analysis of the prostate cancer mortality difference between the two randomized groups was already showing a difference of 20% at that time, favouring the screened group, which passed the pre-set statistical requirements.

Benefits and harms

Both absolute rates of benefit, as well as harm, are clearly presented in the paper. The proportion of subjects experiencing each sort of outcome, per year of follow-up is clearly presented: benefits, in terms of prostate cancer deaths, as well as risks—the side-effects of screening, its subsequent diagnostic work-up, and any treatment provided for screen-detected cancers. The inverse of those proportions is also provided: the' number needed to treat (or screen)' (NNT or NNS—see Chapter 7) in the case of benefit, and the analogous 'number needed to harm' (NNH), which reflects the number of persons experiencing significant harmful side-effects of screening, per clear beneficiary whose life was extended by screening. To the great credit of the 2009 paper, its final discussion (p. 1326) and its abstract provide a clear explication that the NNT/NNS, at that point in the trial's follow-up, was 1,410[28] men requiring to be offered screening, or 1,068 men to be actually screened with PSA, an average of slightly more than twice each over nine years, in order to prevent one death from prostate cancer.

Much more important for decision-making at the policy level for PSA testing, the NNH of men for each clear beneficiary of screening (whose life was extended) is also clearly presented in the ESPRC trial publications: 48 other men had to be told after nine years of follow-up (37 men in the 2012 publication, after a few more years of follow-up[28]) that they had prostate cancer and offered some sort of treatment, for each beneficiary of screening. For those men who actually are treated for screening-detected prostate cancer, with surgery, radiation, and/or chemo-/hormone-therapy, experts estimate that some 20 to 30% end up with serious complications, including impotence and other sexual dysfunction, urinary incontinence, and occasionally bowel problems (US Preventive Services Task Force, 2012b).

In short, the PSA test in this trial failed the usual criteria for screening, not because it did not reduce mortality from the disease in question, it did that, by 20% among all those invited to be screened (indeed, prostate cancer mortality was reduced by 27% among just those men actually receiving the test, but that calculation is not as relevant to planning a new screening programme, since it does not consider the typically imperfect uptake of screening invitations by patients). Rather, PSA carried the highest risk, which has ever been documented in an RCT of screening: at least 33 cases of cancer (in the latest follow-up publication, of 2012) to be notified, counselled, and (in many cases) treated in some aggressive fashion, for each man whose life was lengthened. No other form of cancer screening ever thoroughly evaluated has shown such an unfavourable risk/benefit ratio, involving such clinically serious side-effects.

Comparison of PSA testing with mammography

The NNT/NNS for PSA testing found in the ESPRC may seem large, at about 1,000 persons screened twice over nine years per beneficiary. However, this NNT/NNS is not very different from the NNT/NNS for other widely-accepted cancer screening tests. Mammography in women age 50–69, for example, while saving lives, is similarly rather inefficient, with an NNS of 1,339 for women age 50–59, and 337 for women age 60–69, expressed in terms of the number of well women who have to have a mammogram to prevent one breast cancer death (Nelson et al. 2009). [These are the only two age-groups of women at normal—as opposed to high—risk of breast cancer who are currently recommended by the US Preventive Services Task Force to have regular mammograms.] Similarly, the proportionate risk reduction for breast cancer mortality achieved by screening, across these two age-groups, was found by the USPSTF to be 17% across all those invited for mammography, very close to the 20% found for PSA screening in the ERSPC.

The key difference between these two forms of cancer screening, however, is that the more serious medical harms (unnecessary surgical biopsy procedures that result from both false-positive mammograms, as well as over-treatment of benign lesions detected by mammography) are considerably less frequent than the equivalently serious sorts of harms caused by PSA screening (sexual dysfunction, incontinence, etc.) Published estimates suggest that, during the two decades of biennial mammograms currently recommended for all women age 50–69 by the USPSTF, perhaps 50% will suffer from either a false positive mammogram or over-diagnosis/over-treatment of an essentially benign tumour. Some will require a breast biopsy to determine that the mammogram-detected abnormality is benign; others, subject to over-diagnosis and over-treatment, will be treated regardless. A USPSTF-commissioned mathematical modelling study, Mandelblatt et al. (2009), which used a sophisticated range of assumptions and methods to estimate that, for every 1,000 women accepting the nine biennial mammograms, over the 20-year age-period when the USPSTF recommends them, about 5.4 women (one in 185) would have their lives extended. How do these benefits compare with the harms and how does that ratio compare between mammography and PSA testing? Box 8.2 summarizes and contrasts the harms of PSA and mammography testing.

To summarize, neither screening programme is particularly efficient at reducing cancer deaths. Both cause considerable harms in the process, but PSA testing would appear to carry worse risks, in terms of the magnitude of the NNHs involving the more serious harms associated with both confirmatory biopsies, as well as the very invasive and risky treatments currently available for prostate cancer, even though more and more men with early disease and relatively benign histology are being managed merely by 'watchful waiting'.[29] Much of this difference between the two screening programmes is attributable to their disparate test-positivity rates (16% of men screened by PSA, versus 4% of mammograms recalled for repeat screen and/or biopsy for mammography), and the much higher rate of over-diagnosis (perhaps 50% for PSA-diagnosed cancers, compared to perhaps 20% for mammography-detected cancers.)

The bottom line

To summarize, the ERSPC trial was a landmark in the rigorous evaluation of cancer screening, and a model of how a high-quality screening trial should be conducted. There are weaknesses in the study, for example the

Box 8.2 Comparing the harms of prostate specific antigen (PSA) and mammography cancer screening tests

What are the comparative rates of harms from PSA and mammography cancer screening tests during the recommended period of screening? For mammography the recommended period of screening is every 2 years between the ages of 50 and 69 years (20 years). For PSA testing, although there was no consistent recommendation before the European Randomized Study of Screening for Prostate Cancer (ERSPC, Schröder et al. 2009; Schröder et al. 2012), extending that trial's screening frequency to a non-selective age range of trial eligibility would lead to screening every 4 years between the ages of 50 and 75 years (25 years). Therefore, the figures below are rates per 1,000 people screened for the recommended period; nine mammograms tests over 20 years or seven PSA tests over 25 years. The data discussed here are taken from the ERSPC (Schröder et al. 2009; Schröder et al. 2012) and Mandelblatt et al. (2009).

False positive screening result/unnecessary biopsies

Mammography

780 false-positive mammograms—some of these would be corrected by simply repeating mammograms, often following a period of 'watchful waiting' of borderline abnormalities for a period of months or longer. Such periods are typically very stressful for the patient. This figure translates into a *number needed to harm* (NNH) of 144 (= 780 ÷ 5.4 (NNT or number needed to screen (NNS))) women experiencing a false positive mammogram result that is subsequently found to be inaccurate for each women whose life is extended by mammography.

PSA testing

Although this information is not directly available from the ERSPC trial it can be easily calculated as follows (Schröder et al. 2012):

Positive PSA test rate × Negative biopsy rate = PSA false positive rate

16.7% (167 per 1000) × 14.1% (141 per 1000) = 2.4%% (24 per 1000)

However, this figure only relates to having had two tests, 4 years apart, so it needs to be multiplied by 3.5 (seven tests divided by two tests) to get the total false positive rate for PSA screening over a man's lifetime: 24 × 3.5 = 84 per 1,000.[30] This figure translates into a NNH of 24 [84/(1.07 (NNT/NNS per 1,000 men screened twice in the ERSPC trial) × 3.5)]. Twenty-four men per beneficiary is also an estimate of the lifetime NNH, in terms of 'unnecessary prostate biopsies' per beneficiary, as judged by their having negative findings for cancer. This NNH is smaller than the equivalent number modelled by Mandelblatt et al. for a lifetime of nine mammograms: 55 unnecessary breast biopsies per woman whose life is extended by the screening. However, both these figures are misleading because at least 50% of 'positive' biopsies for 'cancer,' after a positive PSA test (as defined in the ERSPC trial) are now thought to represent *over-diagnosed cancers* of no clinical significance, which require additional NNH calculations.

Over-diagnosis cases per beneficiary (a subset of NNH)

Mammography

About three women over-diagnosed with breast cancer for each life saved, based on a 'best-estimate' of over-diagnosis of 19% of all cancers detected by mammography, calculated for only those women actually undergoing screening (Independent UK Panel 2012).

PSA testing

The comparable figure for the PSA trial at latest follow-up is at least 16 (33 men per death averted who were told they had 'cancer' in the ESPRC trial, multiplied by the >50% estimated over-diagnosis rate) over-diagnosed men per life saved.

heterogeneity of how PSA-positive patients were managed across the seven participating countries. As well it is possible that some of the health benefits in the screened group may have been created not by screening, but rather by systematically better medical care in the academic medical centres where these subjects were cared for, as opposed to the more local, non-academic centres caring for many of the control subjects (Miller 2012). However, on the strength of the ERSPC trial, most epidemiologists, including those sitting on the US Preventive Services Task Force, would not now recommend PSA testing for any men at normal risk of prostate cancer, at any age. Furthermore, there is a practical difficulty with the recommendation that every primary care physician should discuss the pros and cons of PSA testing for asymptomatic prostate cancer. The harsh reality, of high patient volumes in most of the world's general practice surgeries, about six patients per hour in the current NHS, makes that recommendation unworkable. Most patients prefer their doctor to decide on the preventive measures they are given as part of their regular check-up, on the basis of the physician's best scientifically-informed judgement, and knowledge of their particular profile of health risks (including family history of major diseases, as well as 'lifestyle' risk factors). A complicated lecture about the epidemiology of screening is unlikely to clarify decision-making for most patients.[31]

Postscript: so why have regular medical check-ups at all?

The thoughtful reader will have discerned the overall message of Chapters 7 and 8: *caveat emptor* ('buyer, beware') when it comes to preventive medical care for well persons with no symptoms. It can often do more harm than good, and only sometimes leads to attractive NNTs/NNSs, versus NNHs, to achieve long-term health benefits at little risk, often several years in the future.

This is not to advocate that general practitioners stop setting aside time to discuss effective preventive interventions, which are appropriately tailored to each individual's future medical risks. Many studies have shown that physician-supported smoking cessation, and brief physician-interventions to reduce alcohol consumption in those with high intakes, are effective and cost-effective (National Institute for Health and Care Excellence, 2006a, 2010; US Preventive Services Task Force, 2009a, 2013a). As shown in Chapter 7, the assessment of a person's baseline risk of future cardiovascular disease or death is generally useful, even if only to initiate a discussion of readily modifiable risk-factors—e.g. overweight, sedentary lifestyle, low-quality diet—which have been widely accepted as worthy of intervention by the patient, acting after joint decision-making with his/her physician.

Indeed, trained general practitioners in most developed countries are well aware of carefully generated lists of recommended, evidence-based preventive interventions, many of them specific to particular age and gender groups. A clear example is Pap screening in well women; another is blood pressure measurement every half-decade or so in persons without any risk factors for hypertension or other CVD risk factors, and more often when those risk factors are present. This sort of recommendation is especially reliable when it has been produced by independent, inter-disciplinary panels of scientific experts, such as those convened by the US Task Force on Preventive Services, or NICE in the UK. Such bodies have identified and assessed the precise evidence of each preventive intervention's effectiveness and efficiency, considered it transparently, and followed accepted epidemiological and health economic standards for assessing evidence quality, such as those which this book attempts to set out.

Likewise, it is widely accepted that the under-diagnosis and under-treatment of depression (whether by 'talking therapy' or prescription drugs) is perhaps the largest single cause of preventable disability, one now rising rapidly in the world rankings. Depression, and the contributing conditions in the patient's life, some of which can often be modified with great benefit and little risk, is often not detected by busy physicians, nor complained about by patients, unless time is spent discussing broader health risks on a regular basis. One hesitates to call this sort of general preventive appointment by the terms historically most often used—the 'periodic health exam', or the 'health check-up'. However, most health care-providers and many patients have experienced patient benefit from the scheduling of such preventive office appointments on an occasional basis.

Regrettably, recent systematic reviews of RCTs of health checks for well persons, executed over nearly forty years in several countries, have consistently failed to show that even restricting such check-ups to only the most evidence-based content is not a guarantee of measureable health benefits from attending them (Krogsbøll et al. 2012). While there are legitimate scientific criticisms of these studies, e.g. they were mostly too small and short-lived to be able to show subtle, but potentially important long-term benefits of check-ups, one thing about this literature is striking. Despite the best efforts of extremely earnest and skilled investigators, across the 14 high-quality trials summarized by Krogsbøll et al. (2012) spanning publication dates from 1963 to 1999, there is no strong evidence that the more recent, typically better-designed and analysed trials have found any clearer benefits than earlier studies. Furthermore, no overall benefits were found in this meta-analysis for any of the following rather diverse outcomes: total, cardiovascular or cancer mortality; hospitalization, overall morbidity, disability, or worry; savings in physician visits; or reduced absence from work.

Worrisomely, this review did find that regular preventive check-ups did lead to a 20% increase in the number of new diagnoses per patient over six years of follow-up, and a higher prevalence of essentially screening-detected, asymptomatic conditions, such as elevated blood pressure and serum cholesterol levels, with the expected accompanying increase in the prescription of anti-hypertensive medications (most of these trials pre-dated the widespread, aggressive use of statins.) Whether these screening-detected patients with 'silent' chronic disease risk factors, have truly benefited from such long-term treatments, is not evident from the review. As the authors have argued in Chapters 7 and 8, such benefit largely depends on just how aggressively those patients were managed, in terms of the threshold of future disease risk acted on, and the relative risk/benefit profiles of the treatments deployed.

Notably, Krogsbøll et al. (2012) pointed out that enthusiasm for universal health checks, for entire segments of the well adult population, has apparently diminished in recent years—they cite the 'abandonment' of the Danish national programme. However, they note that an essentially similar 'Health Checks' programme in the UK NHS appears to continue to be implemented, albeit implemented more by paying GPs to do specific preventive manoeuvres on a case-by-case basis, rather than paying doctors specifically to perform a less-well-defined 'complete check-up.' Remarkably, however, such check-ups remain the hallmark of expensive private medical care on both sides of the Atlantic, with some 'executive care' clinics even promoting new methods of screening that no respectable expert currently recommends (due to the probable risks, high costs, and dubious benefits involved.) A good example is whole body scans. These inevitably uncover asymptomatic, hidden structural, or functional defects of completely uncertain importance to future health, but which often end up being aggressively treated, 'to play it safe.' The excellent book by American physician Dr Gilbert Welch et al. (2011), 'Over diagnosed' provides many compelling examples of how such un-validated screening, and over-treatment of the 'incidentalomas' that it finds, can do more harm than good.

In short, there is still—despite decades of scientific publications to the contrary—plenty of 'prevention snake-oil' still on offer in the health care systems of the high-income countries. That is, of course, a major reason why the authors wrote this book.

Decision support tool

Evidence assessment—2D and E.

Considering the individual, community, or population perspectives—1, 2, 3, and 4.

Considering your personal perspective—1.

Quiz

The serious reader should try to apply the CASP Critical Appraisal questions for Randomized Control Trials, for which a website URL is listed in Appendix 2, to the 2009 ERSPC paper (Schröder et al., 2009), and then compare his/her answers to those the authors have developed for teaching, which are found in Appendix 3.

Supplementary questions

As described in this chapter the authors have found the CASP RCT appraisal questions to be entirely applicable to screening RCTs. However, the authors have created a few supplementary questions, to bring out the extent to which such a study has: (a) avoided the common biases in evaluating cancer screening; (b) quantified the main sorts of potential harms; and (c) quantified both the clinical efficiency (NNS) and risk/benefit balance (harms per beneficiary—NNH) of screening, as follows:

Question 1: If other health benefits of screening are claimed, e.g. screen-detected cases with less advanced cancers, easier and cheaper to treat, and with a better outcome, do the analyses adequately take account of 'length-(time) bias' and 'lead-time bias' to convince you that they are real benefits, as opposed to, respectively, these two artefacts

1. *'Length(-time)' or 'diagnostic' bias:* screening's inherent tendency to *preferentially* detect very slowly growing cancers, including some which would not normally lead to symptoms in a patient's lifetime, leading in turn to *over-diagnosis* and, potentially, *over-treatment*?

2. *Lead-time bias:* screening's misleading *apparent* capacity to add years to the 'median/mean survival time after diagnosis', and to increase the '% five (or other "n")-year survival after diagnosis', even if cases detected by screening die at the same average age as they would without screening? This occurs purely because earlier diagnosis 'starts the survival clock' at an earlier point in the patient's life, and so increases survival time, independent of any actually increased lifespan. In other words, even if a screening program were completely ineffective in reducing the age-specific/standardized death rate from the cancer being screened for, a five- (or other) year survival improvement would be seen in the screened group, compared to the unscreened group, purely because their tumours were detected earlier by screening, even though the treatment then applied was not able to extend the screened cases' lives at all. This point is almost impossible to get across to lay audiences—with the result that every week the popular press, and many press releases from cancer advocacy groups, but also, sadly, major government reports on cancer survivorship internationally, proclaim that cancer survivorship is either improving, or not, more in one population group than another, entirely on the bogus basis—at least for frequently screened cancers—of five- (or other) year survival rates.

Question 2: Are all the potential harms of screening identified and quantified—or at least acknowledged and discussed?

For example,

1. Additional anxiety and/or depression in those found to be screening-test positive, but who may have to wait weeks or months for the results of confirmatory diagnostic testing (such as tissue biopsy), which are then negative?

2. Screening-induced side-effects of invasive confirmatory diagnostic testing—again, especially in those found to have either no disease as a result, or disease of such benign natural prognosis that its detection leads to over-diagnosis/over-treatment?

3. Screening-induced unnecessary side-effects of over-diagnosis and over-treatment, in this last group who are positive on confirmatory diagnostic testing, but whose disease is unlikely to have ever led to clinical consequences in their lifetimes, if left undetected by screening?

4. Screening-induced 'false reassurance' in persons who actually have prostate cancer, but are screened falsely as normal ('false negatives'), who then delay in presenting with symptoms of the undetected disease, later on, in the mistaken belief that their earlier negative screening test result was 100% accurate?

Question 3: Is the 'clinical efficiency' of the screening program summarized in credible calculations of:

1. **'Number (of persons, over a given number of N years of follow-up) Needed to Screen' ('NNS')** *per clear beneficiary?* = the reciprocal of the difference in the primary outcome rates in the unscreened and screened groups, after screening a specified number of times, over a specified number of years. [It is particularly useful to calculate this as an intention-to-screen—or *effectiveness*—analysis, the number of persons who had to be *offered* the screen for each clear beneficiary, especially if the clinical encounter making this offer required significant resources—for example to explain the potential benefits and risks of screening—and/or led to a relatively low rate of acceptance of screening.] This is a non-valuated (non-economic) measure of screening programme efficiency, and is the first step in calculating its actual cost-effectiveness, but is much easier to compute (in that it requires no cost assumptions) and to understand.

2. **'Number Needed to Harm' ('NNH')?** = number of persons clearly adversely affected by screening (i.e. the sum of those experiencing any of the measured risks of screening already outlined) *per clear beneficiary*. This is a convenient summary of the risk-benefit balance of the screening programme, in that it quickly indicates if there are more 'victims' or more clear beneficiaries, overall.

Chapter 9

Genetic testing for disease prevention: oversold?

Background

Genetic testing is a controversial field and an inherently complex one. Therefore, the authors start with a summary of the basic scientific issues around the contribution of genetic factors—of all sorts—to the major serious diseases of the developed world:

+ Coronary heart disease and stroke.
+ Type 2 diabetes and its major risk factor, overweight, and obesity.
+ The commonest cancers.
+ Dementia.

Taken together, these conditions account for more than two-thirds of premature deaths and serious disability as we move past middle-age. The authors have summarized below the key points about the genetic contribution to these diseases' causation, before moving into the specifics of genetic testing for predicting disease risk. The enthusiastic reader is referred to a substantial book chapter on this topic (Frank et al. 2006b), the arguments of which are still pertinent.

Some basic truths about the contribution of genetic factors to the major diseases of the developing world

The media regularly tout the promise of 'personalized medicine', based on genetic testing to detect DNA markers of future disease risk. However, that promise remains largely unfulfilled. A major reason for this failed expectation is that even multiple DNA markers, corresponding to dozens to hundreds of separate genes or other locations in our long strands of DNA, still only have very modest predictive accuracy for the major illnesses of later life.

Despite daily media reports of new studies claiming to show the strong influence of genes in human health, the truth is that the commonest diseases of later life that drive health care expenditure in the developed world, are influenced at least as much by the environment as by our genes. Frank et al. (2006b) provide specific examples, but even lay persons without formal scientific training are aware that most of these illnesses are not that commonly replicated within a single family tree. A more elegant example is presented in Box 9.1 (Frank et al. 2006b). This example demonstrates that the environments in which we grow up, live, and grow old profoundly influence our risks of common diseases of later life—through our diets, patterns of physical activity, personal habits, and vices (tobacco, alcohol, and drug use, sexual practices, and other forms of risk-taking), as well as exposures to specific toxic substances, energy forms (e.g. radiation, noise, heat/cold, and sunlight), as well as other physical factors, such as altitude or high atmospheric pressures, and infections. Box 9.1 shows how such environmental factors change over time and space, altering the precise effects on our health and function of the specific genes we inherit.

Certain global diseases are entirely determined by the presence of *one defective gene* (so-called Mendelian inheritance, after the nineteenth century Moravian monk, Gregor Mendel, whose clever breeding of sweet peas allowed him to discover the basic principles of modern genetics). In contrast to the dominant cholesterol gene discussed in Box 9.1, many such single-gene disorders cause disease only when both copies of that gene that a person carries are defective (the so-called 'recessive' pattern of Mendelian inheritance). Among the commonest of such diseases are sickle cell disease and other genetic disorders of haemoglobin (the oxygen-carrying protein in our blood), such as thalassemia, while another is cystic fibrosis. However, these 'single-gene disorders' are not nearly as common—at least in most global settings—as the major diseases causing of premature illness and death in the developed world (listed at the start of this chapter). That is because these rare single-gene disorders are so damaging to normal human function that they have been selected against in human populations through human evolution, in that most of them cause greatly reduced reproductive capacity in those affected, at least those diseases that start in childhood. The exception to this rule is disorders of haemoglobin, which are relatively common in entire populations in the tropics—for example, sickle cell disease in much of Africa. In that setting, the sickle cell gene is—in the mild or asymptomatic 'carrier' version called sickle cell 'trait,' due to having only one defective gene, rather than two—actually protective against a major health threat on that continent since time immemorial—malaria. Mother Nature has thus selected for sickle cell trait (the carrier state) through its protective effect against a major killer. However, nature takes back, as the 'price' of that population health benefit, the combination of recurrent severe illnesses, and typically early deaths of those individuals in whom both copies of that gene are abnormal.

Box 9.1 Genes, cholesterol, and mortality over 150 years

In 2001, Sijbrands et al. published an elegant study summarizing the mortality experience, over a period of about 150 years, of hundreds of Dutch citizens in a set of extended family trees. These families were identified from their descendants, who carry a rare, but potentially lethal gene that massively elevates serum low-density lipoprotein (LDL)—'bad' cholesterol levels. Affected persons have historically lived foreshortened lives due to aggressive coronary heart disease (CHD). Until the advent of statin drug therapy about 25 years ago, CHD death in early adult life was common in such families. In affected pedigrees (the blood relatives and ancestors of affected patients), the rate of this condition is expected to be 50%, since the gene is dominant. Remarkably, Sijbrands et al. (2001) were able to track down the birth and death dates of virtually all the relatives, living and dead, of the affected patients they had cared for, stretching back to all deaths since about 1850. [Deaths after 1985 were not analysed, because the advent of statins prevented many early deaths in later generations.] The main finding of this analysis was that the affected family members died, on average, at much older ages in the nineteenth century, compared with their normal countrymen—not at younger ages, as would be expected from the effects of their cholesterol-elevating gene that we observe today. These families' mortality did begin to rise above that of their normal neighbours after World War I, reaching a maximum in the 1950s and decreasing steadily thereafter—precisely in parallel with the rise and fall of CHD mortality in the general population. Sijbrands et al. (2001) hypothesize that the families' defective gene must have originally protected them from early deaths, due to a disease that commonly caused early-life mortality in Europe before WWI, but not afterwards—tuberculosis is the obvious candidate. [TB is thought to have been made less common due largely to improved nutrition, although the jury is still out on that (Catalano and Frank 2001).] In that era, the gene was kept in the Dutch gene pool by natural selection, through these protective effects. Otherwise, families carrying it would have likely died out long ago. However, an equally worthy hypothesis is that some new environmental exposure, widely distributed beginning about WWI, interacted with the gene in question, so as to greatly raise the risk of carriers developing early and lethal CHD, at least until statins became widely available. The graph in the paper strongly suggests that the post-WWI changes in men's and women's mortality, in these families, were separated by about 10–20 years, almost exactly the lag-time between the onset of the two sexes' epidemics of smoking. Other factors may well have played a part, but the study demonstrates that even a normally lethal gene's health effects can be massively moderated by the environment, in ways that can change within a few human generations. The gene did not change, but its health effects did, because those are jointly determined by the environment.

There is a further complication to the process of using genetic markers to predict garden-variety disabling diseases of later life. For these so-called 'complex' diseases, risk is typically contributed to by dozens to hundreds of separate genes, and the complex interactions between them, as well as the multiple environmental exposures of individuals, as they pass through the stages of life, as already noted.[32]

The essentially 'polygenic' nature of the genetic contribution to the causation of the common diseases of later life means that the strength of association between any one gene and one of these diseases is typically quite weak. As explained in Chapter 3, this strength of association is usually summarized in a relative risk (RR) of developing the disease for those with the gene in question, versus those without it. For complex diseases involving a large number of gene and often many environmental causes, RRs of substantially less than 1.5, and often less than 1.1, characterize the usually observed associations between each implicated gene and the disease in question). Those low RRs translate into inaccurate predictive performance when we attempt to use such genes/markers in a well person, to predict serious complex disease many years to decades later. On the other hand, a person with one copy (if the gene is 'dominant') or two copies (if the gene is 'recessive') of a defective gene that causes a single-gene disorder (such as those discussed) is typically very likely—in some cases virtually certain—to develop the disease in question.[33] An example of a complex disease, with polygenic inheritance thought to influence about 30% of the total disease risk, is colorectal cancer (CRC). Box 9.2 explains how even the discovery of many genetic markers associated with CRC has not yet led to their routine use in predicting CRC risk in well persons, even for making decisions about how aggressively to screen for asymptomatic CRC by other, more traditional screening tests.

These challenges to the accurate prediction of common chronic diseases of later life by purely genetic testing, have unfortunately not constrained the commercial sector—especially in America—from offering unproven genetic tests for sale to consumers. These poorly-regulated testing services, often available

Box 9.2 The challenges of using weakly associated genetic markers of disease risk to select high-risk persons for screening— colorectal cancer (CRC)

This common cancer of the developed world has a much better outlook when detected and treated early. However, currently available screening tests suitable for use in the general healthy population (usually over age 50, unless there is a strong family history or other unusual risk factors present) are either:

♦ Imperfect in their ability to accurately detect early disease (e.g. the stool-for-occult-blood test, which may miss as many as half the colorectal cancers developing over the next decade or so, despite its use every few years (US Preventive Services Task Force 2008)

and/or

♦ Expensive and somewhat risky (e.g. sigmoidoscopy and/or colonoscopy to directly visualize the colon and rectum, both of which occasionally lead to bowel perforation, haemorrhage, and/or infection).

Consequently, much recent research has attempted to use genetic markers of CRC risk to identify a higher-risk subpopulation, who would then be offered the more intensive/risky/expensive screening modalities (currently, endoscopy). However, a 2010 paper by a Canadian group of genetic and cancer epidemiologists calculated that 140–160 accurately detectable gene variants, each demonstrating the typically weak association with CRC, indicated by an average RR of 1.2, would be required in order to achieve an arbitrarily defined (but quite sensible) benchmark for discriminating a high-risk subpopulation for endoscopic screening (Hawken et al. 2010). That benchmark is the identification of a subpopulation experiencing 80% of the subsequent CRC cases, but amounting to only 50% of the entire population (in whom full colonoscopic screening would be much more cost-effective than in the general population, due to their high risk). [The rest of the population, at low risk, could then be offered much less intensive and expensive screening, such as the stool test for hidden (faecal occult) blood, since they are at low risk—that test is much less sensitive than colonoscopy, but the substantial fraction of early CRC cases it misses would amount to quite rare events in a low-risk population.] The authors predicted that this large number—140–160—of weak, separate polygenic influences on CRC risk would eventually be discovered, although at the time of writing in 2010, they estimated the current number of genes/markers associated—even weakly—with CRC to number perhaps 80. However, Hawken et al. (2010) are less than enthusiastic about the potential of such purely genetic markers for even improving the efficiency of non-genetic colorectal cancer screening programmes, through the accurate identification of persons at high risk. Their caution, recently reinforced by Chowdhury et al. (2013), stems from the fact that genes/markers with stronger disease associations are the most easily detected epidemiologically, and are thus usually identified relatively early in the history of relevant research. After several years of such research, the stage we are at now for genetic markers of CRC risk, a half-decade after the earlier publication appeared, is such that only new genetic markers with very weak associations (RRs typically between 1.0 and 1.1) continue to be discovered. These weak associations tend, for statistical reasons, to be the most difficult associations to replicate in independent studies, and thus establish as scientifically valid risk factors (Box 3.1). As well, because of their low relative risks, they do not add much to existing risk-prediction algorithms and, therefore, the effectiveness of genetic screening, based on all the markers discovered earlier, which (as already noted) typically have stronger disease associations, on average (Goldstein 2009). In short, there is a problem of 'vanishing returns' from expecting more purely genetic research to lead to better risk prediction for common complex diseases that are polygenic, as well as substantially influenced by the environment. What is needed is the identification and accurate quantification of something much harder to study: gene-environment interactions. [A full discussion of the complex challenges in detecting and characterising gene-environment interactions is beyond the scope of this book; interested readers can access a non-technical summary of the issues, from the point of view of trying to design giant cohort studies for this purpose, in a paper written by a multidisciplinary team of researchers from across Canada (Frank et al. 2006a).]

online, have been shown to frequently provide epidemiologically unvalidated genetic test results, which have either unknown or only limited predictive validity for the subsequent development of the diseases in question. For example, Little and Hawken (from the same Canadian research team) note:

> It is well established that genetic testing for low-penetrance alleles [i.e. gene variants that only occasionally lead to disease and typically carry very small

relative risks of a future disease, typically 1.1 to 1.3—*authors' addition*], one at a time, is not useful in a screening or diagnostic context and may even cause unintended psychosocial harm (Little and Hawken 2010, p. 257).

It is to that potential for harm, from inaccurate genetic testing for future disease risk, that this chapter now turns.

A worked example of the potential risks, as well as benefits, of genetic screening for future disease risk

Classifying the accurate versus erroneous results of any diagnostic or screening test may be achieved by employing a simple tool: the 'two-by-two' table (i.e. two rows and two columns) summarizing test validity results. In an easy-to-read paper by Madlensky et al. (2005) this table is adapted for use in predicting future disease, as opposed to its usual use in diagnosis or screening to detect current disease (Chapter 8). This adaptation merely consists of relabelling the two column headings, from those used to assess the validity of diagnostic/screening tests to detect disease already present ('Disease actually present' and 'Disease actually not present'), as shown in Table 9.1:[34] [See the CASP website, http://www.casp-uk.net, for a tool using these concepts, to critically appraise studies of diagnostic tests, which is not a focus of this book.]

To clarify, 'a' is the number of persons tested who have the genetic (or other) marker of future risk, and eventually do develop the disease, within a specified period of follow-up. 'b' Is the number of persons tested who have the marker,

Table 9.1 Two-by-two table for a prognostic test to predict future disease risk

| | | Future outcome | | |
		Subsequent disease occurrence	No subsequent disease occurrence	Total
Test result now	Positive	a = true positives (TPs)	b = false positives (FPs)	(a + b) = all positive results
	Negative	c = false negatives (FNs)	d = true negatives (TNs)	(c + d) = all negative results
	Total	(a + c) = All future cases	(b + d) = All future non-cases	(a + b + c + d) = n = total number of persons tested

1. Total future incidence of disease, among all those tested = $(a + c)/n$ (within a specified period of follow-up).

2. Total proportion of positive tests, among all those tested = $(a + b)/n$.

but do not develop the disease. 'c' Is the number of persons tested who do not have the marker, but do develop the disease, while 'd' is the number persons tested who do not have the marker and do not develop the disease. Obviously, any persons in cells 'a' and 'd' are receiving correct predictions from the testing, whereas those in cells 'b' and 'c' are being given erroneous predictions. As has long been established in the context of *screening* well persons for *concurrent* asymptomatic disease (Chapter 8), it is also the case in testing for *future* disease prediction that persons in the latter two categories, so-called false-positives (FPs) and false-negatives (FNs), can only be harmed by being tested.

Some persons in the erroneous-result (FP and FN) cells of Table 9.1 in particular FNs, suffer only what may seem a relatively minor harm—not having their future disease occurrence identified by the test (which is merely the equivalent of not being tested at all). Such a FN result could, however, have significant consequences if the patient interprets the genetic test results as 'false reassurance' and then does not follow proven guidelines for reducing the risk of that disease in all patients, regardless of genetic make-up. This could, for example, happen because the patient believes the test result has given them a licence to live as they like—in this case, eating a low-fibre diet with much red meat (known risk factors for CRC), and foregoing useful CRC screening tests, such as colonoscopy. In contrast, those in the FP cell of Table 9.1 might suffer a different sort of harm, in that they may be advised to comply with *completely unnecessary, long-term* actions to reduce their apparently elevated future disease risk, or—if there is no known means of prevention—to at least plan for the elevated possibility of contracting the disease in question. These actions will be pursued by compliant FPs when, in fact, they are not destined to experience the disease at all. There can be more immediate harms for a FP. For example, one of the commonest health-damaging consequences of receiving a positive test for the risk of a future disease that is widely feared, such as dementia, is reactive depression, and the dysfunction and social isolation that often accompany it. Such reactions, while important to treat and understandable in true positives (Table 9.1), are all quite pointless when one's test result is a FP. Both FPs and FNs are victims of *iatrogenesis*.

A substantial scientific literature has grown up around the experience of persons carrying single-genes that very strongly predict future illness, notably Huntington's chorea. Huntingdon's slowly disables those affected, starting in mid-life or earlier, but there is currently no effective treatment. The poignant writings of persons from affected families, who have been able to obtain accurate genetic testing for many years now, show that there is a significant proportion of sufferers' family members who have decided, after fulsome genetic counselling and due reflection, not to have the test at all. (Huntingdon's Disease Society of America 2016). [The condition is caused by a dominant gene, so half of all related family members are typically affected, eventually, as was the case for the cholesterol gene discussed in Box 9.1.] These test 'refuse-niks' reason that it is not worth knowing in advance that one's life will be foreshortened by a disabling and potentially socially-stigmatizing disease (it causes uncontrollable motions, and so is very socially challenging). This is a compelling argument, given that there is no known way to delay the disease's onset or reduce its rate of progression. As well, concrete harms from such testing can occur if the results of the test are entered into a patient's medical records, then included in any 'required documentation' as part of a subsequent application for life or health insurance (or even mortgage insurance in some jurisdictions). The applicant may sign the insurer's usual consent form, to access all his or her medical records, without even considering the consequences. Furthermore, If the genetic test in question is not well known to physicians or the insurer has little expertise in its interpretation (highly likely for new genetic tests), then insurance options may be restricted or 'rated' at a higher premium because of the positive test result, even if it turns out later to be FP.

What about the potential benefits from being a true positive or negative (cells 'a' and 'd' of Table 9.1)? Madlensky et al. (2005) argue that persons in the 'true positives' category (cell 'a'—TPs) may theoretically experience reduced uncertainty and anxiety, especially if they are tested for the future risk of a condition that has been common in their family, as in the case of Huntington's. Furthermore, if an intervention exists—either medical or self-imposed—to reduce the risk of succumbing to the condition, delay its age of onset, or modify its subsequent rate of progression, having a true positive (TP) test result will improve the benefit/risk ratio of that treatment, and might even lead to increased motivation to comply with that treatment, especially if that treatment is difficult, unpleasant, or expensive.

As for persons in the 'true negatives' (TN) category, they could experience only one sort of benefit—reassurance to allay pre-test anxiety and fear, due to the possibility of the disease affecting them in the future. This is a reasonable benefit to ascribe to testing, if that fear was itself reasonable. For example, such fear is entirely understandable when a person has a strong family history of the health condition in question, for which the future risk is being assessed. Such reassurance is not a credible benefit to claim for testing if the patient has no particular reason to fear the condition because of increased risk assessed on purely clinical grounds (e.g. based on family history), once these facts are explained to him or her. A more subtle risk from TN test results, especially for conditions common in families, is 'survivor guilt,' the negative reaction to being spared, when others whom one loves are not.

The point of this entire discussion, however, is that genetic tests to predict the future risk of complex diseases have final disease outcomes that are *as yet unknown for any individual patient*, at the time when the test result is delivered to the patient. Instead, all the clinician has to communicate to the patient is a set of probabilities. These probabilities are ideally based on long-term follow-up of a large cohort of persons tested at baseline, to ascertain which of them, with which specific test results actually develop the disease or not—precisely the dataset required to fill in Table 9.1. In other words, without the benefit of hindsight, the clinician and the patient only have a genetic test result—'abnormal' or 'normal'—which is *associated with* particular probabilities of future disease. This leads to an inherently uncertain situation, which remains uncertain until cases of the disease actually declare themselves, as the years pass—hardly a recipe for successful 'personalized medicine.'

Let us now calculate some typical future disease probabilities for various test results—in this case for the combined set of then-validated (Madlensky et al. 2005) genetic markers for future risk of colorectal cancer (CRC). We'll use two separate two-by-two tables, one for testing 1,000 patients in the general, low-risk population, and one for testing 1,000 patients in a high-risk population with a strong family history of CRC. The resulting numbers are sobering (see Table 9.2).

Table 9.2 Predictive validity of genetic testing, per 1,000 persons tested for mutations related to CRC risk: (A) in a low-risk, general population; (B) in a high-risk subpopulation with a strong family history of CRC

(A) General, low-risk population			(B) High-risk subpopulation (with a very strong family history of CRC)		
	Later disease occurrence (lifetime)	No later disease occurrence (lifetime)		Later disease occurrence (lifetime)	No later disease occurrence (lifetime)
Test result positive	True positives (TPs) = 1	False positives (FPs) = 1	**Test result positive**	True positives (TPs) = 50	False positives (FPs) = 50
Test result negative	False negatives (FNs) = 49	True negatives (TNs) = 949	**Test result negative**	False negatives (FNs) = 150	True negatives (TNs) = 750

Adapted from *Journal of Clinical Epidemiology*, Volume 58, Issue 9, Madlensky, L et al., 'Risks and benefits of population-based genetic testing for Mendelian subsets of common diseases were examined using the example of colorectal cancer risk', pp. 934–41, Copyright © 2005 Elsevier Inc., with permission from Elsevier, http://www.sciencedirect.com/science/journal/08954356

To summarize these test results, the four-fold increased lifetime risk of CRC in the high-risk subpopulation—(50 + 150)/1,000 = 20%, versus (1 + 49)/1,000 = 5% in the general, low-risk population—has a major effect on how many persons tested end up in each of the four cells of the table. Specifically, the proportion of persons at distinct risk of being worse off with testing than without it (FNs and FPs) is four times higher, at (150 + 50)/1,000 = 20% of those tested, in the high-risk population than in the general, low-risk population, at (49 + 1)/1,000 = 5%. However, this undesirable result in the high-risk setting, comes with a potential benefit for 50 times more tested persons in the TP category (50 per 1,000, versus 1 per 1,000) than in the general population—*if, that is, an effective CRC risk-reducing intervention is available and complied with*—for example, a low-red meat, high-fibre, largely vegetarian diet, perhaps combined with colonoscopy every 5–10 years (US Preventive Services Task Force 2008).

Because only 1 per 1,000 persons screened this way has a clear potential benefit, there is little merit in using the genetic markers available in 2005 to predict CRC risk in the general population. The ratio of likely beneficiaries to potential 'victims of testing', is too small, with a ratio of only 1 TP to 50 persons with erroneous test results (49 FNs and 1 FP). In the high-risk population, on the other hand, that ratio is made more attractive, not only by the 50-fold greater proportion of TPs, but also by the greater probability that the TNs actually benefit from 'valid reassurance', since their strong family histories probably carry with them entirely reasonable pretest angst about their future CRC risks.

The message here is, as with so many forms of testing for disease that is not currently causing clinical symptoms or signs in the patient—either because the disease is still at an early and silent stage (e.g. cancer screening, Chapter 8), or because it will not develop for some years into the future (e.g. risk factor modification, Chapter 7, and CRC genetic testing)—*the most effective and efficient use of preventive testing and treatment is among high-risk populations.* This fundamental principle, emphasized in both Chapters 7 and 8, is underscored here, again, for testing for the risk of future disease by genetic markers.

What then is the problem?

The difficulty with the calculations shown are that they require the skilled clinician's application of his/her up-to-date knowledge of a disease's clinical, laboratory, and genetic risk factors. This knowledge depends on being aware of the findings of all relevant, high-quality cohort studies of that disease. This is rather a tall order in the modern world, due to the rapid rate of publication of such studies, scattered across hundreds of research journals internationally—ergo the importance of recently updated Systematic Reviews and Practice Guidelines (Chapter 4). The skilful clinician uses that knowledge, together with facts about each patient, to estimate that patient's 'pre-test likelihood' of any future disease of concern. The pertinent facts about the patient constitute their risk-factor profiles. These profiles can usually be gleaned—as was seen in the case of cardiovascular disease risk assessment in Chapter 7—from a simple history (including family history), physical examination, and non-genetic laboratory tests, such as blood cholesterol or sugar levels. Many of the commonest chronic diseases, such as coronary heart disease, stroke, and Type 2 diabetes, can be quite accurately predicted with just this common risk-factor information alone. In these circumstances, the added value of newer genetic tests is often limited, in terms of predictive accuracy, especially for complex diseases such as these, which have multiple genes and environmental factors contributing to their causation. In the hands of well-trained physicians, nurse-practitioners, and genetic counsellors, this more traditional risk-assessment, without specific genetic testing, is typically adequate for an informed decision to be made, by patient and caregiver together, about the usefulness of additional genetic testing—including its risks.

On the other hand, direct-to-the-public marketing of largely unregulated genetic tests, as is common now in North America, is another matter entirely. It is unethical at best, because it leaves the innocent patient (and his/her family, where genetic marker tests are concerned) alone with the inherently complicated decision of whether to do the genetic test or not, without reliable and independent advice on the relative risks and benefits.

The ongoing failure of regulation of the American medical self-testing market, with its internet tentacles throughout the world, stands as a clear example of unacceptable preventive practice. It is almost certainly doing more harm than good. On other hand, it is quite profitable for the firms involved. In a damning indictment of such commercial practices, Janssens et al. (2008) published a thorough critique of the typically low predictive accuracy, and the attendant risks and costs, of a standard 'personalized medicine' package of diverse genetic marker tests then available in the USA. They found that many of the genetic markers detectable with the expensive packages then on offer had never been properly validated, through replication in more than one epidemiological study of high quality. In other words, it is not even clear that these markers have a clinically significant association with the subsequent occurrence of the disease in question. The average consumer could not possibly be expected to discern which such genetic tests are valid, and which are truly likely to confer more benefit than risk. The situation today is not any better, in that a sophisticated mathematical modelling study of whole-genome sequencing did not predict the risk of the most twenty-four common diseases, including Type 2 diabetes, cancers, stroke, and coronary heart disease (Doerr and Eng 2012; Roberts et al. 2012). The current US Federal Trade Commission (2014) website clearly warns consumers considering the purchase of genetic testing. In the UK, a 2012 Report by the Parliamentary Office of Science and Technology (2012) also railed against under-regulated and oversold direct-to-consumer genetic tests. *Caveat emptor ...*

To conclude, the authors offer a quote from the final paragraph of JFs 2006 book chapter on 'Interactive Role of Genes and the Environment,' which is as valid now, 10 years on, as it was then:

> The determinants of most common diseases are complex, with environmental and genetic/biological factors interacting over the life course, embedded in a social context. Focusing exclusively on the genetic strand of this intricate web of causation—although profitable for some—will not address many other important disease determinants . . . There are forces in our society . . . pushing for a purely genetic approach to ill health, and this means we are at risk of using genetic technology in an inappropriate and unbalanced way . . . However, if we can achieve an appropriate and balanced use of new genetic technologies, we will improve our understanding of how genes and the environment interact to cause many common diseases. Such a goal would in the spirit of Rose's maxim[35] to 'seek the causes of incidence' in populations, rather than simply the 'causes of cases' among individuals (Frank et al. 2006b, p. 28).

Text extract reproduced from Frank, J et al., 'Interactive role of genes and the environment', in Heymann, J., et al. (eds), *Healthier societies: from analysis to action*, Oxford University Press, New York, USA, Copyright © 2006, by permission of Oxford University Press USA.

Decision support tool

Evidence assessment—2D and E.

Considering the individual, community or population perspectives—1, 2, 3, and 4.

Considering your personal perspective—1.

Quiz

In the traditional '2 by 2' table depicting the validity of diagnostic or screening tests for disease that is already present in the patient's body, the proportion 'a/(a + b)' in Table 9.1 is termed the 'positive predictive value' (PPV) of the test: the probability that an abnormal ('positive') test result correctly identifies the presence of the disease in question. In genetic testing for the future (typically lifetime) risk of a disease, that proportion is sometimes linked to a long-used genetic term, 'penetrance', which refers to the capability of a genetic trait to manifest as a disease or other actual outcome in a person's body. However, traditional use of this term in genetics has sometimes implied that penetrance is a rather fixed biological property of a given genetic trait. Epidemiologists, on the other hand, know from Bayes' Theorem (Porta 2008, p. 16) that PPV is not at all fixed, but rather algebraically dependent on the proportion of the tested population that actually has the disease in question—(a + c)/(a + b + c + d)—the disease's prevalence in that population. [That is why the PPV is always helpfully higher in higher-risk populations.] However, the discerning reader will have realized that the analogous fraction in the genetic test validity table is, in fact, the future cumulative incidence of the disease in the tested population. Can you see how that incidence would vary across different cohort studies attempting to estimate the values of all four cells in Table 9.1, for a given genetic marker of future disease risk? What could be done to make the calculation of penetrance more standardized? [For a discussion of this question, see Madlensky et al. (2005).]

Chapter 10

When can prevention expect to also reduce social inequalities in health?

A brief overview of social inequalities in health

French and English medical officers were among the first to tabulate rates of death across different geographic areas, and groups of citizens, within a city, county or country. Louis-Rene Villerme (1782–1863), and his near-contemporary, Marx's close friend Frederich Engels (1820–95) used mortality rates, a fundamental tool of what was to become the science of epidemiology. These rates were used to quantify discrepancies in longevity across age groups among the labouring classes, in contrast to the educated and the gentry. Villerme's most famous work on the subject (1839) declares:

> The excessive mortality among families of workers employed in the cotton spinning and weaving mills in Mulhouse mainly affects the younger age groups. In fact, one-half of the children born to the class of manufacturers, businessmen, and factory managers reach the age of 29, whereas one-half of the children of weavers and factory workers in the spinning mills will die, as hard it may seem to believe, by age 2 (Villerme 1839, as cited in Buck *et al.* 1988, p36).

Since the nineteenth century, a number of generalizations—*axioms*—about such socio-economic *gradients* in health outcomes have been found to hold across remarkably diverse societies, through long historical periods:

Axiom #1

Socio-economic gradients in health virtually always show a steady worsening of health outcomes as socio-economic status (SES) declines, in a stepwise fashion: Thus, while the health of the poor is worse than that of the rich (with few disease exceptions), it is striking that the health of the middle class is nearly always mid-way between that of the two most-extreme social groups. Indeed, incidence and mortality rates for the commonest diseases in most societies show extraordinarily detailed step-functions across ten or more rank-ordered levels of SES[36]—as Fig. 10.1 illustrates for premature (below age 75) all-cause mortality in Scotland. This aspect of such gradients has a further corollary: most cases of illness or death that represent an 'excess attributable to sub-optimal SES' (i.e. rates of adverse health outcomes above those seen in the most privileged groups) are found in the large majority of modern populations at 'middling' SES levels, not among the poor per se. This is simply because the middle classes are more numerous than the poor in more 'economically developed' societies (though not, it should be noted, in the world's poorer countries).[37]

In turn, this corollary implies that policies or programmes intended to reduce health inequalities have to reach, and change health status among, the middling classes. Sir Michael Marmot—perhaps the world's foremost authority on health inequalities for the last quarter century—has repeatedly pointed out (Marmot 2010; UCL Institute of Health Equity 2014; World Health Organization 2008) that the policy-language equivalent of this inference is that *universalist* policies directed at the whole population are critical to reducing health inequalities. Since some additional policy focus on the most needy is often also required, Marmot refers to the most promising policies as exhibiting 'proportionate universalism' (Marmot 2010; UCL Institute of Health Equity 2014; World Health Organization 2008).

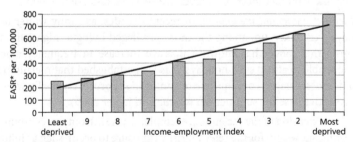

Fig. 10.1 All cause mortality amongst those aged <75 years by Income-Employment index: Scotland 2012 (European Age-Standardized Rates (EASR) per 100,000).

Reproduced from The Scottish Government, Statistical Bulletin: Health and Social Care Series, An Official Statistic Publication for Scotland, *Long-term Monitoring of Health Inequalities: Headline Indicators*, October 2014 Report, © Crown Copyright 2014, under the Open Government Licence v.3.0., available from http://www.gov.scot/Publications/2014/10/7902/downloads#res461784

Axiom #2

SES inequalities in health status are typically seen across a wide spectrum of physiologically diverse diseases and injuries, in terms of their underlying causes. Using the annual Scottish Reports on Health Inequalities again (Scottish Government 2014), all eleven health outcomes analysed show the same direction of association with SES: the wealthier and more educated a Scot is, the better his/her health outcome, on average. 'Inverse' health gradients do exist in the industrialized world, for a small number of conditions where specific life-course exposures make the privileged more affected than the poor. Examples of inverse socioeconomic gradients in health include;

♦ *Allergies (including hay fever—allergic rhinitis and conjunctivitis—and asthma)*, hypothesized to occur more frequently among the privileged (in some settings) because human beings need a degree of exposure to less than perfectly hygienic conditions as they grow up, in order for their immune systems to develop—the so-called 'hygiene' hypothesis, still under investigation (von Mutius 2007).

♦ *Incident breast cancer* (although not generally mortality from this condition), largely because the reproductive lives of women at lower SES levels have historically included more pregnancies, starting at younger ages. These reproductive risk factors all contribute to lower breast cancer incidence in less educated and less privileged women, partly due to their reduced exposure over the life course to the strong hormonal female hormonal fluctuations of the menstrual cycle: the fewer such cycles in a woman's lifetime, due to late menarche, more pregnancies, or less time lactating, the lower her risk of breast cancer (US Preventive Services Task Force 2009b).

♦ *Incident malignant melanoma*: in recent decades, as sunny winter holidays were taken up among the more privileged living at high latitudes, this lethal cancer has shown a massive increase in frequency among those able to afford such holidays. It is well established that melanoma is a decades-delayed consequence of sun over-exposure, especially with no protective baseline summer tan (Garbe and Leiter 2009).

♦ As an extension of the melanoma example, any health outcomes requiring significant wealth for the relevant risky exposure to occur, such as injuries from potentially dangerous and costly sports (alpine skiing, scuba diving, equestrian events, sky-diving, etc.). However, deaths due to these causes, while potentially important for the wealthy constitute a very small proportion of all deaths in modern societies.

Many scientific observers have suggested that this protean, or medically non-specific, effect of SES arises from a biological mechanism by which SES affects health (Hertzman et al. 1994). Various kinds of deprivation alter our high-level regulatory processes (related to our *physiological stress responses*) that link our daily experiences, over a lifetime, to the function of both our immune and endocrine systems—these regulatory processes are the 'orchestra conductors' of the mind-body (Hertzman and Frank 2006).

Axiom #3

Overall health inequalities (for example, as summarized by life expectancy or all-cause mortality rates) by SES tend to be remarkably persistent in a given population, across decades or longer, even though the specific medical causes of illness, injury, and death have changed (Evans et al. 1994). If all sorts of daily stressors adversely affect our health through non-disease-specific biological pathways, then the plethora of stressful life events at low SES levels will manifest as worse levels of health status in that social group, no matter what illnesses are currently predominant in a society. As an example, in most of Europe in the nineteenth and early twentieth centuries, the commonest cause of death in early adulthood through mid-life was tuberculosis (TB). Accordingly, TB exhibited a strong social gradient in Europe, whereby the poorer classes suffered it more frequently.[38] Then, over a century after the mid-1800s, TB incidence declined precipitously throughout Europe, even though virtually nothing was known about is microbial cause until the 1880s, or its effective treatment until the 1940s, when the first antibiotic able to kill the TB bacillus, streptomycin, was discovered (McKeown 1976). Yet European social gradients in mortality have persisted at similar relative[39] levels over the last several decades (Mackenbach et al. 2015), even though the major causes of death in Europe have gradually shifted. For example, coronary heart disease and stroke have greatly declined; cancers of various sorts have become either more or less frequent, overweight/obesity and its major complication (Type 2 diabetes, and its complications in turn) have become much more common; dementia and its complications appear to be more common (although that may be mostly an artefact of older populations), and motor vehicle accident deaths have come down substantially.

Much recent research has examined possible reasons for this remarkable capability of SES inequalities in health to perpetuate themselves for long historical periods, even when the diseases of society—and indeed, the risky exposures and behaviours predominant in society—change greatly. Most social epidemiologists now think this is due to a second mechanism, above and beyond daily stressors acting on diverse body systems through 'master control panel' pathways such as psycho-neuro-immunological and psycho-neuro-endocrine ones (Hertzman and Frank 2006): the embedding of such stressors' effects on our body-mind function over the life-course. The first few years of life especially provide opportunities for such 'embedding'. Ground-breaking cohort analyses of David Barker in the UK, and Clyde Hertzman in Canada, show that many common diseases of later life have their risks powerfully set in early life. Furthermore, some of those risks are unlikely to be fully reversible, despite personal avoidance of 'lifestyle' risk factors that tend to become long-term habits in the teens and early adulthood, such as smoking, poor-quality diet, a sedentary lifestyle, and excessive alcohol consumption (Hertzman and Wiens 1996).

A good example of early life embedding of late-life disease risk is dementia, including Alzheimer disease. More than one study has shown that the onset of clear symptoms in this condition is substantially delayed in persons who have completed more formal education in their youth, or who demonstrate early-life evidence of a high intellect. A widely publicised analysis of the written essays of young nuns, kept safely until the authors were elderly and some of them demented, showed that the more complex a demented nun's written expression was in her youth, the later she showed the first symptoms of dementia (Riley et al. 2005). Other studies suggest that each level of additional basic education (primary, secondary, post-secondary) is associated, on average, with about a half-decade of delay in the onset of the common dementias. This is much less true of the rarer premature dementias, which tend to have a strong genetic basis, presumably because the genetic factors that tend to drive early-onset dementia swamp out the 'environmental' influences of basic education (Reitz et al. 2011). Some dementia experts believe that the relative protection afforded by educational attainment is due to the more complex wiring connections in the brains of more intelligent and better-educated persons (Katzman 1993). Such 'brain reserve' presumably enables these patients to continue to function longer, as the disease process progressively interrupts more and more of the rich connections between their neurons. It has also been suggested that dementia's downhill course, towards major disability and death, is paradoxically much more rapid in more educated and intelligent patients, simply because the disease is advanced when it first causes symptoms; however, a recent structured review of that evidence did not confirm a worse prognosis for Alzheimer disease in more educated patients (Paradise, Cooper and Livingston, 2009).

In recent years, social epidemiologists have noted that the commonest diseases of later life—sometimes referred to as 'diseases of comfort' (Choi et al. 2005)—have become just the opposite in most post-industrial societies: diseases concentrated among the disadvantaged. Many studies have shown that the less privileged tend to suffer more frequently from later life conditions, and more prematurely, than the privileged do (Marmot 2010; Marmot et al. 2008). Furthermore, that pattern can only partially be attributed to the widespread tendency for low-SES populations in developed societies to smoke more (though not necessarily to drink more alcohol; Marmot 1997), eat less nutritiously, exercise less, and in general 'behave badly' (Lynch et al. 1997). Some observers use these facts to 'blame the victims'. This view supports policies that tend to appeal to individual responsibility on the part of ordinary citizens to reduce chronic disease risk factors among both deprived and non-deprived populations. However, studies from the social and behavioural sciences point to the sizeable commercial apparatus in place in all western democracies to influence lifestyle 'choices', through ubiquitous advertising and marketing practices (Lang and Rayner 2007; Moodie et al. 2013; Stuckler et al. 2012). Public health experts increasingly recommend state-sponsored as well as consumer-collective intervention to change the incentives around these lifestyle choices. Exemplary policies include the subsidization of healthier foods, drinks, leisure-time physical activities, and active transport, as well as higher pricing and more regulated availability of tobacco, alcohol, and 'junk foods' (Capewell and Graham 2010; Dahlgren and Whitehead 2007; McGill et al. 2015; Frank et al. 2015). There is some evidence, to which the authors now turn, that such public health interventions, while not always popular, are precisely those most likely to reduce health inequalities by social class.

What sorts of preventive interventions are likely to reduce inequalities?

This book has advocated the critical appraisal of scientific evidence on the effectiveness of prevention. So why not just use systematic reviews of existing intervention studies, of the highest quality, to generalize about, which preventive interventions are most likely to have favourable effects on health-equity and, which ones to be cautious of, in that they may increase health inequalities by SES? Unfortunately, very few public health programme and policy intervention studies to date have *properly assessed potentially differential health impacts, according to the social class of persons* targeted by the intervention (Lorenc et al. 2013; Tugwell et al. 2010). Indeed, even the relatively well-research area of preventive tobacco control has as yet only a small number of high-quality studies addressing differential impacts by SES (Hill et al. 2014; Ogilvie et al. 2008).

Part of the reason for this dearth of evidence, on all sorts of health (and other) sector interventions' impacts on health inequalities by SES, is technical: to assess such differential impacts of a policy or programme can be onerous and expensive, in terms of study design and particularly sample-size (Tugwell et al. 2006; Welch et al. 2012). There is also something of a tradition in medical research to simply ignore such differential impacts, and assume that—since most summary measures of *clinical* interventions' effectiveness are expressed as *relative risk reductions*—health interventions should automatically lead to greater absolute benefits among persons at lower SES, who typically have the highest baseline health risks (Anderson et al. 2005). However, in the case of public health interventions, or policy interventions aimed at the broader social determinants of health, there is widespread agreement that because such interventions are generally 'complex'—in both their design and their impacts (Craig et al. 2008)—their effectiveness tends to exhibit marked sensitivity to local cultural and social context, including differential health impacts by SES. Thus there have recently been strong calls for better-quality evaluations of such intervention's impacts on health inequalities by SES (Craig et al. 2011).

As an interim remedy to the current shortage of empirical evidence on the impact of public health and preventive interventions on health inequalities, Sally Macintyre, former Director of the MRC Social and Public Health Sciences Unit in Glasgow, has assembled a thoughtful list of the broad characteristics of policy, programme, and public health practice interventions most likely—as well as those most unlikely—to reduce health inequalities by social class (Macintyre 2007). Box 10.1 summarizes those excellent criteria, with an example of each (provided by the authors).

In the last four cases in Box 10.1 the potential for a preventive intervention to only *reach* as far as the privileged is clearly evident; in the first four, as many potential barriers to universal participation/compliance have been removed as possible—for example, via governmental or third sector subsidy. As well, some of these examples relate to the well-known tendency for the best-educated, and those with the most disposable income and freedom with their time, to participate most actively in any new trends, as 'early adopters' (Rogers 2002).

Among the sorts of preventive interventions listed in the first half of Box 10.1, many public health experts have recently come to believe that the best single investment of 'social and community resources' for reducing health inequalities by social class in any society—is *proportionately universal, high-quality early child development and education programmes* (Hertzman et al. 2010; Keating and Hertzman 1999; Marmot 2010; Nores and Barnett 2010; Temple and Reynolds 2007). Analysis of Program for International Student Assessment (PISA) 2009 data has shown that increasing the duration of high-quality early childhood 'education and care' (ECEC) to more than one year, among pre-schoolers across the UK would have resulted in a 20-point increase in the UK's PISA literacy test scores in youth, and a world-ranking among countries, which would be 12 places higher (Mostafa and Green 2012). Modelling the impact of universal

Box 10.1 Examples of public health (and preventive) interventions that are more likely, and less likely, to effectively reduce health inequalities

More likely to reduce health inequalities:

- Structural changes to the environment, legislation, regulatory policies, fiscal policies: e.g. legislation to remove trans-fats from foods sold in restaurants or stores (as opposed to informational campaigns urging consumers to demand this change in food composition).

- Income support: e.g. a 'living wage' minimum wage law (typically focused on the public sector, where more support is commonly found), as opposed to an employers' voluntary programme to pay at least this wage.

- Improving accessibility to public services: e.g. free bus passes for the elderly, those on benefits and the disabled (as opposed to case-by-case issuing of passes only upon application, and passing a rigorous set of eligibility tests).

- Prioritising disadvantaged population groups, through intensive support, and starting young: e.g. universal free entry to neighbourhood drop-in Early Child Education/Development Centres (as opposed to requiring formal membership application or means-testing).

Less likely to reduce health inequalities

- *Written materials*: e.g. pamphlets (as opposed to radio/TV/social media messaging—because the latter assume no literacy barriers to understanding)

- Campaigns reliant on people taking the initiative to opt in e.g. requiring written and mailed application to participate (as opposed to simpler means of joining—e.g. via social media)

- Whole-school health education approaches to smoking and alcohol use: e.g. posters and intercom announcements (as opposed to bespoke and more interactive messaging to particular groups at risk)

- Approaches that involve significant out-of-pocket costs or other potential barriers to participation: e.g. *fitness programmes requiring paid membership in health clubs (as opposed to no-cost programmes located in local community/drop-in centres)*

Adapted with permission from Macintyre, S., *Inequalities in health in Scotland: what are they and what can we do about them?*, Medical Research Council (MRC) Social and Public Health Science Unit, Occasional Paper No. 17, October 2007, Copyright © MRC SPHSU 2007, available from http://www.sphsu.mrc.ac.uk/publications/occasional-papers.html

ECEC on children's PISA literacy scores has also shown a major reduction in score variation across the full range of parental social class (Mostafa and Green 2012). This tendency has earned ECEC the label 'win-win' policy, because it 'boosts average performance and reduces inequalities' (p. 22). Economists call this a 'Pareto improvement' (Culyer 2005), and there are not many of them in the modern policy-maker's kitbag.

The challenge, of course, is that not all societies enjoy wide political and cultural acceptance of the view that 'everyone needs to support (and pay taxes to support) proportionately universal early childhood education and care.' Some societies tend to see the responsibility for providing such care as falling entirely to individual parents and families. The classic graphs of PISA scores—in maths, and as well as language skills—consistently show the 'fan' pattern seen in Fig. 10.2 across two decades of research (Willms 2003).

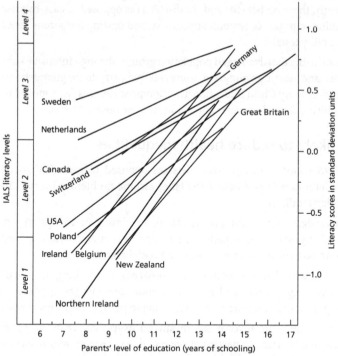

Fig. 10.2 Socioeconomic gradients in standardized literacy test scores by parental education level (selected countries, 1990s).

Reprinted from *International Journal of Educational Research*, Volume 39, Issue 3, Willms, J.D., 'Literacy proficiency of youth: evidence of converging socioeconomic gradients', pp. 247–52, Copyright © 2004 Elsevier Ltd., with permission from Elsevier http://www.sciencedirect.com/science/journal/08830355

That pattern contrasts societies with the more universalist view of early childhood education and care (epitomized by northwest continental Europe), showing the smallest gaps between the educational attainment levels of children born to educated versus uneducated parents—with societies, epitomized by the USA, with more individual-responsibility embedded in their views on this matter, which show the largest gaps. From the point of view of the unborn child, one could say that 'when selecting where you want to be born into this world,' it matters little to your eventual educational accomplishment, and therefore your lifelong wages and economic success (on average—for the graph only depicts averages), which sort of family—educated or uneducated—you are born into, as long as you are born in the former sort of country (e.g. Scandinavia or the Netherlands). However, it matters a great deal what sort of family you are born into if you enter the world in one of the countries whose data in Fig. 10.2 and in more recent analyses showing precisely the same overall pattern show steep gradients in PISA scores against parental education. Surely compassionate societies should not leave matters such as the fairness of educational outcomes by SES to the vagaries of chance. Proportionate universalist ECEC policies, as well as equivalently pro-equity and redistributive policies throughout any country's educational system, at all levels, are one of the most important policy levers available to reduce economic, social, and health inequalities, throughout the life-course.

Conclusion

As implied in Chapter 5, in our discussion about the challenges of evaluating interventions that act at the level of entire societies, rather than individuals, it remains very challenging for public health researchers to provide concrete advice to policy makers regarding, which preventive interventions at the societal level are most capable of reducing health inequalities. To reiterate, this challenge is partly related to the technical difficulties of designing and executing robust evaluations of the effectiveness of such policy and programme interventions, which are often impossible to randomize to large numbers of population groups. Notwithstanding that challenge, our multi-disciplinary group at the Scottish Collaboration for Public Health Research and Policy recently published a summary of what they regard as the best 'investments' any modern society can make to support health equity over the life-course (Frank et al. 2015). We also analysed in that paper the extent to which these policies have been successfully implemented in recent years in Scotland, as opposed to England and Wales, and how much effect we could find, in terms of expected changes SES inequalities described by routinely collected health, education, and economic statistics. These 'Seven key investments for health equity over the life course' are summarized in Box 10.2.

The authors appreciate that some of these best investments are contentious, and many of them politically and logistically, as well as economically, very challenging to act on. However, on the strength of all the evidence we could find, we believe that they constitute the best advice that public health researchers can currently provide policy-makers, at least in the UK, about how to reduce health inequalities by SES in the future.

Box 10.2 Seven key investments for health equity across the life course

◆ *Investment #1*: universally accessible (free at point-of-care), strongly promoted, high-quality sexual and reproductive education/counselling in youth; family planning; prenatal and perinatal care.

◆ *Investment #2*: labour market, tax and transfer policies to lift all families with young children out of poverty.

◆ *Investment #3*: universally accessible (virtually free), high-quality early childhood education and care programmes, located in every neighbourhood within walking distance of parents' homes.

◆ *Investment #4*: systematic support to enable universal secondary and—where appropriate—post-secondary—education and training, suited to full and productive employment.

◆ *Investment # 5*: accessible (free at point of care), high-quality primary, secondary and tertiary health care, combined with evidence-based public health services

◆ *Investment #6*: strong, evidence-based economic and marketing controls on established health hazards, including: tobacco, alcohol, unhealthy foods, and gambling.

◆ *Investment # 7*: green policies for sustainable and equitable economic development, including full, meaningful employment.

Decision support tool

Evidence assessment—2B, C, and F.
Considering the individual, community or population perspectives—1, 2, 3, and 4.
Considering your personal perspective—1.

Quiz

Immunization, especially if a high level of population coverage is reached across a whole society, is usually regarded as a quintessential example of a public health preventive intervention that can reduce health inequalities of any sort. Childhood vaccination programmes in well-managed public health systems often achieve this goal. However, vaccines given during adolescence and adulthood are much more likely to reach smaller proportions of the socially marginalized, including low-SES groups, ethnic minorities, etc.— partly because they involve more 'voluntary' participation on the part of individuals consenting to be immunized. The current state of HPV vaccination against cervical cancer (and, for some vaccines, genital warts and other related cancers) has achieved widely varying coverage rates among per-teen girls since it was introduced in wealthy countries nearly a decade ago. What would you anticipate would be the sorts of health inequalities created by low HPV vaccine uptake in some social groups? [*Answer*: For a full discussion of this issue, and some mathematical modelling of possible health inequalities from low HPV vaccine coverage, see Crowcroft et al. (2012).]

Postscript

This book has attempted to inform the reader about the intelligent and critical analysis of claims made for prevention—not only when he/she is a 'patient' (even a well one) in a health care system, but as a citizen in a community, where unsupported claims of effective prevention also abound.

The authors hope that the conceptual and technical tools offered will assist our readers in being critical about prevention, whether one is demanding 'truth in advertising' in a doctor's office, a community council meeting, or at the ballot-box. Using these tools to point out the lack of credibility of some claims of preventive effectiveness—made on behalf of various personal actions, community programmes, and societal policies—may make one rather unpopular. If one uses these tools to suggest that the intervention in question may do more harm than good, one may be even less popular. However, one will be a more effective patient, citizen, and person as a result.

Appendix 1

Preventive actions: decision support tool

Evidence assessment

1. *Assess existing summaries of relevant scientific knowledge:*

   (A) *Evidence identification.* Have you searched for and retrieved any relevant evidence summaries, in particular systematic reviews of the effectiveness/benefits/risks/costs of the proposed preventive intervention?

   (B) *Evidence quality assessment.* Have you critically appraised those evidence summaries using recommended tools?

   (C) *Overall assessment.* Is the evidence, as summarized in existing structured reviews, of sufficient quality to inform your decision? If so, stop evidence assessment here and move on to 'Considering the individual, community or population perspective'. If not, proceed to section 2 immediately below.

2. *Assess evidence from 'original-studies' for and against intervention effectiveness and efficiency:*

   (A) *Causation studies:* Does the evidence demonstrate a causal link between the factor to be prevented and the outcome (e.g. disease)? [This step may be skipped if step 2 (D), below, has been addressed by high-quality, relevant studies.]

   (B) *Relevant category of prevention:* Does the evidence favour primordial, primary, secondary, or tertiary prevention? [The answer should guide the search for studies to address the last two questions below.]

   (C) *Relevant 'Rose-ian' prevention strategy.* Does the evidence favour individual- or population-level preventive actions? [Again, the answer should guide the search for studies to address the next two questions below.]

   (D) *Overall effectiveness.* What information do existing high-quality studies provide regarding *all* the effects of the preventive intervention's (benefits, harms, costs)?

(E) *Overall efficiency*. What information do existing high-quality studies provide regarding the relative attractiveness of the resource investment required to implement the intervention, given its benefits and risks, compared with other competing uses of the same resources to improve health?

(F) *Equity considerations*. Does the preventive intervention under consideration fall into any of the eight categories listed in Box 10.1, which are likely to either increase or decrease health inequalities, especially those by socio-economic status?

Considering the individual and community/population perspectives

1. *Relevance*. Is the available evidence relevant to you as an individual or the community/population you are concerned about (external validity)?

2. *Burden of illness*. What is the risk and relative severity of the disease in individuals like you, or like the population you are concerned about?

3. *Justification for action*. Does the risk and severity reasonably support the use of potentially more harmful or intrusive preventive actions to avert it (i.e. when examined by a person of 'reasonable judgment')?

4. *Overall feasibility/acceptability*. Is the preventive action feasible and acceptable to you as an individual, or to persons in the population you are concerned about?

Considering your personal perspective (especially for health professionals)

1. *Your bottom line*. From your personal perspective, given all of the above, would you take the preventive action? Would you recommend it for the patient or population you are concerned about? Why (or why not)?

2. *Alternative actions*. Does your knowledge, expertise, and experience suggest any other potentially effective, efficient, feasible, and acceptable preventive actions for the health outcome in question, not considered in the evidence assessment thus far?

3. *Assessing the alternatives*. What could you do, with the help of others if necessary, to gather evidence which would support your new preventive action?

Complete this process for each alternative preventive action.

The authors would like to hear your views on this tool:

- How helpful did you find this to be?
- What sorts of situations and settings would you consider using it or have you used it in?
- Are there any changes you would suggest to improve it?

Please send your responses to the senior author: john.frank@ed.ac.uk.

Appendix 2

Useful resources for a critical appraisal tool kit applied to disease prevention

How to critically appraise cohort studies of associations implying causation

The UK-based Critical Appraisal Skills Programme 'CASP' (http://www.casp-uk.net/) provides an easily useable and free critical appraisal tools for assessing all the main study designs referred to in this book, as well as helpful guidance on their use. The tool for appraising cohort studies can be found at: http://media.wix.com/ugd/dded87_e37a4ab637fe46a0869f9f-977dacf134.pdf

How to critically appraise case-control studies of associations implying causation

Again, the authors recommend the CASP website tool for case-control studies: http://media.wix.com/ugd/dded87_63fb65dd4e0548e2bfd0a982295f839e.pdf. [If the reader is not already familiar with the case control design, the authors recommend any introductory textbook of epidemiology, such as Hennekens et al. (1987, chapter 6, pp. 132–52).]

How to critically summarize multiple studies of disease causation (especially for the effects of environmental exposure)

As presented in Box 3.1, the authors like the critical appraisal questions derived from the original causation criteria of Bradford Hill by Gee (2008).

Assessing the methodological quality of systematic reviews

The authors prefer the AMSTAR checklist for this purpose, the use of which is illustrated in Table 4.1: http://amstar.ca/

How to critically appraise non-RCT

In order to critically appraise non-RCT (i.e. quasi-experimental/observational) studies of the effectiveness of preventive interventions (especially those implemented at the level of whole communities/populations, such policy or regulatory/legislative change).

The authors recommend a set of critical appraisal questions created by our colleague Sally Haw (University of Stirling), which the authors have found helpful in teaching (these are found at the end of Chapter 5).

How to critically appraise economic evaluations (including cost-effectiveness studies)

As referred in Chapter 7, the authors recommend the CASP critical appraisal checklist for assessing such studies, although some reading in a basic text of health economics (e.g. Drummond 1997) may be needed for those new to this field: http://media.wix.com/ugd/dded87_3b2bd5743feb4b1aaac6ebd-d68771d3f.pdf

How to critically appraise RCTs of screening programmes (especially for cancer)

As described in the Quiz question at the end of Chapter 8, the authors have found the CASP RCT appraisal questions to be entirely applicable to screening RCTs.

However, the authors have created a few supplementary questions, to bring out the extent to which such a study has:

♦ Avoided the common biases in evaluating cancer screening.

♦ Quantified the main sorts of potential harms.

♦ Quantified both the clinical efficiency (NNS) and risk/benefit balance (harms per beneficiary—NNH) of screening.

These are found at the end of Chapter 8.

Appendix 3

Suggested answers for quiz questions at end of chapters

Chapter 2

Question: Suggest an example of an anti-obesity programme/policy for each of the categories of prevention introduced in this chapter, as a hierarchy—primordial, primary, secondary, and tertiary. Which of your exemplary interventions has, in your view, the most potential traction, and which have the least, in terms of the widespread support across society that would be required in order to implement it?

Suggested answer: For a formal analysis of potential control measures for obesity, all of them aimed at either primordial or primary prevention, and based on the 'ANGELO' framework, see: Mooney J et al. (2015). Note that these measures do not include the more clinically orientated secondary prevention (screening for the early stages of obesity and treating those cases) or tertiary prevention (case-finding full-blown obesity cases and treating those.) All these measures have a role, but without significant efforts being placed on primordial and primary prevention, the regular creation of new cases, in each birth cohort as it ages, will continue unabated.

Further reading

Mooney, J., Jepson, R., Frank, J., and Geddes, R. (2015). Obesity prevention in Scotland: policy analysis using the ANGELO framework. *Obesity Facts*, **8**, 273–81.

Chapter 3

Question: In the USA over two decades ago, a new and frequently fatal disease began to strike down women of reproductive age, after only a short illness: 'toxic shock syndrome' (TSS). Pathology and clinical studies suggested that the culprit was a bacterial toxin absorbed into the body from a mucous membrane. However, because the condition was so rare (only some dozens of cases had occurred when the first epidemiological study on causation was done), a cohort study was not appropriate; only a case control study (Appendix 2) could identify potential risk factors for the condition. This study clearly suggested that use of a particular brand of menstrual tampon was the exposure that led to TSS (Todd et al. 1978). In fact, because the study found that *all* the TSS cases had used the implicated brand of tampon, compared with only 26% of the healthy controls, the estimated relative risk (strength of association) between this exposure and the outcome TSS was effectively infinity. However, the absolute risk of acquiring TSS, related to the use of that brand of tampon, was very small, suggesting that there must have been other key factors operating besides use of the implicated tampon brand that combined to cause the disease. What do you think may have been the legal arguments used by the lawyers acting for the manufacturers of this tampon, in defending their clients from civil litigation brought against them by TSS victims and their families? How would you respond?

Suggested answer: This comprehensive review of the entire TSS epidemic in the USA reveals that several other risk factors, besides the use of a specific tampon brand, contributed to the causation of the TSS in more than 1,400 cases in this national outbreak. Legal counsel for the manufacturers accused of culpability could be expected to exploit this multifactorial pattern of causation by arguing that exposure to more than just the high-risk tampon brand itself was necessary for clinical cases to develop, i.e. such use appears to have been a necessary, but not sufficient condition for TSS to occur. In some legal settings, this would not be deemed convincing legal evidence of causation.

Further reading

Reingold, A.L., Hargrett, N.T., Shands, K.N., Dan, B.B., Schmid, G.P., Strickland, B.Y., and Broome, C.V. (1982). Toxic Shock Syndrome Surveillance in the United States, 1980 to 1981. *Annals of Internal Medicine*, **96**, 875–880.

Chapter 5

Suggested answers: Critical Appraisal Questions for Non-Randomized/ Quasi-Experimental Evaluations of Intervention Effectiveness
Note: all page, figure, and table numbers cited below refer to those in the original publication being critiqued (Pell et al. 2008)

Question 1: Did the study ask a clearly focused question?
Suggested answer: The aim of the study is reasonably clearly set out at the end of the introduction (p. 483). 'Our aim was to prospectively compare the number of admissions for acute coronary syndrome (ACS) before and after

implementation of national legislation, overall and according to smoking status'. However, the population has to be inferred from abstract (p. 482) and method (p. 483).

Were the population, intervention, and outcomes clearly defined?

♦ *Population*: people living within the catchment of nine Scottish hospitals (>3 million).

♦ *Intervention*: Implementation of national smoke-free legislation.

♦ *Primary outcome*: Change in total number of emergency admissions to nine Scottish hospitals for ACS between T1 (June 2005–March 2006) and T2 (June 2006–March 2007); and change in numbers of ACS admissions within smoking status sub-groups.

♦ *Secondary outcomes*:

   ♦ *In non-smokers*—change in geometric mean (GM) cotinine (bio-marker of secondhand smoke (SHS) exposure in non-smokers) and self-reported exposure in last 7 days (location and duration).

   ♦ *In smokers*—change in cotinine (bio-marker of tobacco consumption) and self-reported tobacco consumption.

Note: Cotinine is the proximal metabolite of nicotine and is, therefore, a tobacco-specific biomarker of both tobacco consumption and SHS smoke exposure. It can be measured in most body fluids—blood products, saliva and urine. A number of assays are available for measuring cotinine. In this study, samples were analysed using the gold standard method. There are accepted cut-offs for active and passive smoking.

GM cotinine (sum of log cotinine/n) is used for *non-smokers* because of extreme left skew in the distribution of the untransformed data. Cotinine values for active smokers are normally distributed and no log transformation is necessary.

Question 2: Was a quasi-experimental design appropriate?

Suggested answer: The national smoke-free legislation was implemented across Scotland on the same day and so was not amenable to evaluation using a randomized controlled trial (RCT) or certain other non-RCT designs, such as the staggered time-series ('stepped wedge') design. The quasi-experimental design used—a before–after study with a control population (England) observed during the same time period—was therefore the next best design possible.

Note: In some countries, such as Canada, legislation has been implemented on a province-by-province basis over the last 3 or 4 years. It would therefore be technically possible to devise a rolling programme of research, using provinces where legislation had not yet been implemented as controls.

Could an RCT have been conducted to assess the impact of the intervention under study?

In Scotland, however, even had it been feasible to randomize or roll out implementation in different Local Authority (LA) areas (which it would not have been), contamination (for example, people living in intervention LA, but drinking in pubs and/or working in control LA) would be a potential problem.

Question 3: What are the key features of the quasi-experimental design used in this study?

Suggested answer: The key features of the study design were:

A prospective multi-centre before and after study

This would include baseline data collected June 2005 to March 2006, and post-legislation June 2006 to March 2007.

There were two sorts of controls:

- *Control 1*: an historical control showing the underlying trend in Scottish ACS hospital admissions in the 10 years prior to legislation.

- *Control 2*: a geographical control, such as changes in ACS hospital admissions in England between June 2005–March 2006 (baseline) and June 2006–March 2007. Smoke-free legislation was not introduced until July 2007 (pp. 483–4).

Note: The baseline period ran right up to the day before the legislation came into effect. However, a small number of pubs (for example, those in the Wetherspoon chain) had gone smoke-free in advance of the legislation.

On the other hand, some studies conducted in other jurisdictions found that compliance with smoke-free legislation was not immediate and therefore baseline was redefined in those studies to include a 6-month post-implementation period, after which the legislation was judged to have 'bedded in'. Both early implementation and late compliance with legislation would result in a reduction in effect size (this is equivalent to pre-post design equivalent of contamination).

In Scotland, however, compliance with the smoke-free legislation was immediate and high and has been sustained 3 years post-legislation. In a study of bar workers, Semple and colleagues (2007) found an 86% improvement in air quality 2 months post-legislation and an 89% reduction in GM cotinine (2007) in a cohort of bar workers 1 year post-legislation. There was also a 39% reduction in GM cotinine in representative samples of non-smoking adults and children in the general population (Akhtar et al 2007; Haw & Gruer 2007).

What were the primary outcome measures?

For the intervention population: standard case definition for acute coronary syndrome (ACS) (emergency admission, chest pain, raised troponin (biomarker of myocardial damage) in admission blood sample (or second sample if taken within 12 hours of admission following negative troponin on admission blood). Patients with raised troponin due to co-morbidities such as renal failure, but were judged by other diagnostic criteria not to have an acute coronary event, were excluded.

For historical and geographical controls: change in incident acute myocardial infarction (AMI) (ICD10 code 121) was chosen as the best control outcome measure. However, it is not directly equivalent to admissions for ACS as defined in the prospective study. Unstable angina was, by definition, included in the prospective study, but not in the controls. This was because raised troponin was not a criteria for use of ICD10 code 120.0 (unstable angina) until 2007. Incident AMI admissions (ICD-10 code 121) were, therefore, the 'cleanest' outcome measure for the controls.

To test the comparability of data, study patients were linked to SMR01 database and strikingly only 51% had an ICD10 code 121 in the first study period and 52% in the second study period. This highlights the limitations of studies using retrospective routine hospital admission data (p. 490).

What were the secondary outcome measures?

Assessments of SHS exposure in intervention population: in addition to self-reported SHS exposure (location and duration), in confirmed non-smokers, cotinine was regarded as an objective measure of SHS exposure in the last 3–4 days (half-life of cotinine 16–20 hours).

Note: The rapid 'wash-out' of cotinine levels, after reduction in SHS exposure, was critical to its being suitable for use as an intermediary outcome measure in this before/after evaluation design.

How were subgroups defined in the intervention group?

Objective ascertainment of smoking status in intervention population: admission blood samples were tested for cotinine, the proximal metabolite of cotinine. In serum the lower cut-off for active smoking is >12 ng/ml. Smoking status was based on self-reported status and serum cotinine. Self-reported non-smokers with cotinine >12 ng/ml serum were defined as smokers. In confirmed smokers, cotinine was regarded as a measure of recent tobacco consumption.

What other study designs have been used elsewhere to address this question?

Since 2004 there were, as of a few years ago, a number of studies (13 published) that have used routine hospital admission data to assess the impact of legislation. A number of different designs have been used.

♦ Before and after study with geographical control.
♦ Before and after study without geographical control.

- Time series analysis with geographical control.
- Time series analysis without geographical control.

Early studies have tended to have focused on small geographically isolated communities, while more recent studies have looked at much larger populations. There are some important limitations to most of these studies, which limited the conclusions that can be drawn. All relied on retrospective data and the use of clinical diagnostic labels, which may not have been consistently applied either between clinicians or over time. Only one study had individual-level data on SHS exposure and only two had data on smoking status.

Question 4: Were the analyses appropriate and clearly presented?

Suggested answer: The methods of data analysis are clearly described (p. 484) with the primary outcome of the study is presented as a percentage reduction in total admissions (relative risk reduction) for ACS and reductions by smoking status. In addition, sex by age subgroup analyses were conducted (table 1 in Pell et al. (2008)). The method of calculating the confidence interval (CI) intervals around the percentage reductions is clearly described.

Note: It was not possible to estimate change in incident ACS as catchment population denominators were not available for subgroups of the population classified according to smoking status (p. 484). Therefore, numbers of admissions was used as an outcome (one can safely assume denominator populations did not suddenly change over the months before and after March 2006, although one cannot obviously not say the same for smoking and non-smoking population denominators at risk of ACS hospitalization—indeed, the paper estimates the reduction in smoking prevalence 'attributable' to the legislation as 2.3%—see next paragraph). However, a rather sophisticated statistical argument is, however, provided for the use of numbers of admissions as the primary outcome (by Pell et al. 2008, p. 484)—most readers would be forgiven for trusting the *New England Journal of Medicine* to have had properly qualified statistician reviewers ensure this argument is valid!

Studies from other jurisdictions indicate that we might expect a small absolute reduction (say of 1 or 2 percentage points) in smoking prevalence associated with the legislation. This would reduce the total number of smokers and increasing the number of ex-smokers in the study catchment area. The authors argue that this would lead to an under-estimate of reduction in incidence in *former* smokers, but have no impact on incidence rate in *smokers*. As the number of those who have never smoked, in the age group under study, will not have changed over the course of 1 year, the proportionate reduction in numbers of hospitalizations among those who have never smoked equates to the proportionate reduction in incident ACS (p.484).

Question 5: Are the results clearly presented?
Suggested answer: Yes

Patients included in the study

Information on the proportion of patients providing written consent, refusal and unable to participate is provided and is the same in both data collection periods (p. 485). In both study periods a very high proportion (87%) provided informed consent for follow-up with only 5% refusing to participate at baseline and 6% post-legislation. Ethical approval was obtained to extract data from case notes for patients who died after arrival in hospital.

Primary outcomes

The primary outcomes of reductions in relative risk for the total population, smoking status and age sex subgroups (Table 1 in Pell et al. (2008)) are clearly presented. The authors report a large 17% relative risk reduction in ACS associated with implementation of smoke-free legislation. This compares with an average underlying trend of a 3% reduction per annum in first-time admissions for ACS in the 10 years prior to the legislation. The maximum reduction of 9% for any year (2000) is also reported. The reduction in ICD10 121 admissions in England over the same time period as the study was 4%.

RR reductions of 21, 19, and 14%, respectively, are reported for those who have never smoked, former smokers, and current smokers (table 1 in Pell et al. (2008)). [It is useful to remember that this smaller 'effect-size' of the legislation in smokers, expressed as a proportionate reduction in baseline risk, reflects the smaller, but still surprisingly large, marginal effect of SHS in a smoker, presumably due to particular cardiac toxicants in side stream smoke. Furthermore, the much higher ACS risk in smokers means that this only slightly reduced proportionate risk reduction, compared with non-smokers, might still translate into a larger absolute risk reduction.] A total of 67% of the reduction involved non-smokers.

Secondary outcomes

Data on SHS exposure are reported including duration and location of SHS exposure in the last week and GM cotinine. In non-smokers, significant reductions in self-reported exposure in public places—at work, in pubs, and in other locations, but not in private places, e.g. own home, homes of others (table 2 in Pell et al. (2008)). GM serum cotinine in never-smoker ACS patients also fell post-legislation by 18% (p. 487), but this was not as much as 42% reduction seen in equivalent age group in the general population.

Among smokers admitted to hospital with ACS there was no reduction in either mean serum cotinine or mean reported numbers of cigarettes smoked.

Question 6: is the interpretation of findings appropriate?
Suggested answer: The authors conclude that the introduction of legislation in Scotland was accompanied by an overall 17% reduction in ACS hospital admissions, and that the results of the study are consistent with findings from other primary studies and meta-analyses.

Are the findings biologically plausible?

In addition to a relationship between active smoking and coronary heart disease (CHD), epidemiological data has clearly demonstrated a causal relationship between SHS exposure and CHD. However, the relationship between smoke exposure and CHD is non-linear, with heavy SHS exposure conferring the same risk as light active smoking. Chronic active and passive smoking promote both atherosclerosis and plaque development. In addition, there is now a growing body of evidence from studies involving animal models and healthy volunteers that demonstrate the acute effects of SHS, including epithelial dysfunction, increased oxidative stress and increased platelet aggregation.

Are the findings consistent with the proposed mechanisms of the legislation?

There are, therefore, a number of potential mechanisms in which the legislation might impact on hospital admissions for ACS.
In non-smokers the legislation has led to:

♦ Reduced SHS exposure.
♦ In the longer term, reduced initiation into smoking.

In smokers, the legislation has led to:

♦ Possible reduced tobacco consumption.
♦ In the longer term, increased quitting (reduction in smoking prevalence).

As noted earlier, other findings from the national evaluation indicate a large reduction in SHS exposure in non-smokers (both bar workers and the general population), and a reduction in tobacco consumption and increased quitting in smokers (both bar workers and the general population). There was no evidence of displacement of smoking into the home, but rather an increase in self-reported home smoking restrictions.

Is there any evidence of selection bias?

There is no evidence selection bias. The population living within the catchment areas of the nine hospitals was large (> 3 million) and did not change significantly over the study period. ACS admissions to study hospitals accounted for 63% (baseline) and 64% (post-legislation) of Scottish ACS hospital admissions.

Is there any evidence of loss to follow-up or differential follow-up (or inclusion)?

1. Standard definition of ACS was applied in all hospitals.

2. There was no evidence of differential inclusion of ACS patients admitted to hospital. In both study periods, informed consent was obtained from 87% of patients, with no difference in proportions consenting, refusing to participate, and unable to consent.

3. People who died in the community before reaching hospital were lost to follow-up, but deaths in the community were taken into account in the interpretation of the results of the study

Are the control groups and their outcome measures appropriate?

The use of geographical and historical controls is appropriate. However, the outcome measures used for the intervention population (standard ACS definition) and historical and geographical controls (ICD10 code 121) are not directly equivalent. Nevertheless, these control outcome measures were the best available and the large effect size observed is consistent with much other research.

Are alternative explanations of findings ruled out?

Two alternative explanations are considered.

1. A decrease in hospital admissions might have been accompanied by an increase in the number of sudden ACS deaths in the community. However, examination of Registrar General's Office (RGO) data revealed that over the two study periods there was a 6% reduction in deaths in the community due to ACS (codes not supplied; p. 484)

There are two potential confounding seasonal factors—differences in the same months' temperature, and incident influenza between the before and after study periods 1 year apart, which could have affected the results of the study. Both high and low temperatures, and high rates of influenza are also associated with an increase in ACS admissions. Neither temperature nor incident influenza were controlled for in the analysis, however, a month-on-month comparison of admissions revealed that the reduction became more pronounced over time suggesting that neither temperature differences nor differences in incident influenza in the pre and post legislation periods are likely explanation of the total observed effect.

Acknowledgements

Source: data from Pell et al., 'Smoke-free legislation and hospitalizations for acute coronary syndrome', *New England Journal of Medicine*, Volume 359, Number 5, pp. 482–91, Copyright © 2008 Massachusetts Medical Society. All rights reserved. Available from http://www.nejm.org/doi/full/10.1056/NEJMsa0706740

Chapter 5 quiz questions and answers reproduced courtesy of Sally Haw, Professor of Public and Population Health, University of Stirling, UK.

Chapter 7

Question 1: What is that NNT, across the entire period of follow-up reported here?

Suggested answer: Since the number needed to treat (NNT) is calculated as the reciprocal of the difference in risk between the treatment and control arms of a trial, in this case, NNT to prevent one case of minimum cognitive impairment (MCI) over the entire trial follow-up period, by a Mediterranean diet with extra nuts = $1/(0.126–0.071)$ = approximately 18.

Question 2: What is the NNT expressed in the more informative format of 'number of person-years of treatment required for the prevention of one MCI case.

Suggested answer: Since the trial's average follow-up period, across all subjects, was 4.1 years, then the number of person years required, on average, to prevent one case of MCI through a Mediterranean diet with extra nuts = $18 \times 4.1 = 74.5$.

While the former number (NNT of 18) seems rather attractive, especially for a 'natural' dietary treatment that is probably quite safe, the latter number (NNT in person-years of 74.5) reminds us that the diet needed to be taken for an average of over 4 years before these benefits were seen, and presumably would need to be a lifelong diet if one wanted to continue to benefit at advanced age.

Chapter 8

Suggested answers: Critical Appraisal Skills Programme (CASP) Randomized Controlled Trial checklist.

Note: All page, figure and table numbers below refer to those in the original publication being critiqued (Schroder et al. 2009).

Question 1: Research question clarity

Suggested answer: Yes—the research question addressed in this large seven-country RCT is clearly put: 'Does prostate specific antigen (PSA, a blood test) screening, every four years on average, reduce prostate cancer mortality in healthy European men, aged 50–74 years—50–69 years in the 'core group' for all countries—at the start of the programme, over an average of 9 years of follow-up?'

Question 2: RCT/other design appropriateness
Suggested answer: Yes—the participants were properly randomized—the strongest study design for studying screening programmes' *efficacy/effectiveness*, after representative selection from general population lists.
Note: An unusual feature of the design was that those in three countries were randomized before individual consent was provided by each participant, which addresses the useful question 'What is the *effectiveness* of offering this screening programme to an entire population?', since in the group randomized to screening it includes all those subjects who never, in fact, participated (i.e. refusers).

Subjects in the other four countries were randomized only after agreeing to participate, with full informed consent, which addresses the quite different, but also useful question: 'What is the *efficacy* of this screening programme among subjects who actually were screened, at least once? The latter risk-reduction in the primary outcome will always exceed the former (if screening has any such benefits, that is), partly because the former includes refusers not screened at all, and partly because these subjects typically do worse on all health outcomes—the so-called '(healthy) volunteer bias.'

Question 3: Method of allocation and randomization success
Suggested answer: Yes, although no 'blocking' or stratification of subjects accompanied the randomization—for example, by age—Table 1 (p. 1324 in Schroder et al. (2009)—shows that the mean and median ages of the randomized groups were comparable, and the text indicates (p. 1321, middle right) that comparisons of the two groups for causes of death other than prostate cancer, which should be identical, showed that they were. Although data on comparability of the two groups for other variables, such as social class or family history, are not reported, proper randomization should create approximately balanced (equivalent) distributions of all variables important to the primary outcome, including those not yet known to science, especially when the number of individuals randomized is so large (182,160 in this case!)

Question 4: Blinding
Suggested answer: No, but ... Blinding of subjects and caregivers was not done, but it *could not be done* for this type of intervention, since screening leads to invasive biopsy procedures in those found screen-positive. These procedures cannot ethically be done in a 'sham' way in control subjects not screened, since they carry distinct risks (e.g. multiple needle

biopsies of the prostate can lead to haemorrhage or infection). However, the outcome—prostate cancer specific mortality—is so 'hard' and so objectively ascertained in settings such as modern-day Europe (a data monitoring committee ensured that this was so, in both screened and unscreened groups), that experts would not be concerned that a psychological 'placebo' or 'attention' effect could lead to a systematic reduction in that hard outcome's risk, of the size (20% in this trial) that was being sought.

Question 5: Contamination/losses to follow-up/completeness of reporting/intention-to-treat (i.e. screen) analysis
Suggested answer: Yes. All of the participants appear to be fully accounted for in the analysis. For example, Figure 1 and Table 1 (p. 1321 and 1322, in Schroder et al. (2009), show the flow of patients in both screened and unscreened groups, in considerable detail. Furthermore, the primary outcome analysis was explicitly done on an 'intention to screen' basis, as is recommended for such trials, since it includes all subjects randomized to be offered the intervention. As already noted a sub-analysis was done for the four countries where only subjects who had already given consent were then randomized, allowing the calculation of the efficacy of screening among those who actually had it (rate ratio 0.73—a slightly larger 27% risk reduction, compared with the effectiveness analysis showing a 20% risk reduction—as predicted previously). The method of analysis used—a form of survival analysis—optimally utilizes the precise individual follow-up times of all subjects, reflecting the full period during which they are still being regularly assessed for occurrence—the primary outcome, including appropriate 'censoring' of those who died of another cause, or left study before that outcome occurred, or of all subjects who reached a pre-set final date of follow-up for the entire study (31 December, 2006). This approach allows for proper handling of modest losses to follow-up, but these are likely to have been minimal in this trial for another reason. All the participating countries have sophisticated *population-wide cancer registries*, which would be expected to detect the occurrence of, as well as death by, cancer of any participant still living in those countries, even if he left or was lost to the study for some reason.

There seems to be no explicit mention of 'contamination' (also called 'cross-over' between the arms of the trial) in the paper, i.e. the number of subjects who were randomized to the control group, but who ended up having PSA screening anyway (i.e. as this became more widely offered over the decade of the trial, despite the lack of evidence at that time, it does more good than harm!). However, the general rule is that any contamination only reduces the observed difference between the randomized groups' outcomes, so that the observed difference is, therefore, a conservative estimate of what might have been 'achieved' by screening without any contamination (both in a good sense—prostate mortality reduction—and in the 'side effects of screening' sense—see below.)

Question 6: Equivalency of follow-up and data collection in both groups
Suggested answer: Yes—the paper is convincing in this respect, in that it reports identical average and median follow-up times for subjects in the two arms of the trial (mean 8.8 and median 9.0 years, respectively— p. 1325, upper left, in Schroder et al. (2009)). The paper also reassuringly describes arm's length 'data and safety monitoring' by an expert committee, to ensure that the handling of all methodological issues met international standards.

Question 7: Study sample size (statistical power)/follow-up adequacy
Suggested answer: Yes. The pre-hoc power calculations for the study are clearly described (p. 1323, lower left, in Schroder et al. (2009)) and appropriate. They indicate that the study was powered to detect, with a probability of 86%, the 'minimum effect-size of interest,' in terms of prostate cancer mortality reduction.
Note: >80% is the usual recommended probability of detection of such benefits, but RCTs of interventions for which 'benefits absolutely must not be missed', in clinical or policy terms, may be powered for detecting benefits with a 90% probability. However, this higher power demands more subjects/ follow-up time and, therefore, is more costly.

The 'minimum effect-size of interest' was set at a 25% reduction (the usual benchmark for costly and invasive cancer screening programmes, i.e. the minimum benefit generally considered to always be worth detecting) in the risk of prostate cancer-specific mortality (the 'primary outcome'). Finally, this risk reduction had to be statistically significant with a Type 1/ alpha error of 0.05 (after appropriate adjustment for earlier 'peeks' at the data, as is usually recommended for sequential analysis of trials, which is performed when such trials would ethically have to be stopped, if either arm showed clear-cut worse outcomes, before full planned follow-up had occurred). That power calculation was for the initially planned follow-up through 2008. In the event, follow-up was apparently stopped 2 years early (December 2006), no doubt because the data and safety monitoring committee felt that the observed 20% risk reduction (based, again, on a conservative intention-to-screen/effectiveness analysis) was statistically significant: $p = 0.04$. In general, any trial which finds a statistically significant effect did not in practice have an 'inadequate power problem', although it is important to ensure that no improper analyses were done to deal with inadequate power—that is not an issue here.

Question 8: Appropriateness of method of presenting primary outcome results and nature of those results

Suggested answer: No concerns—as noted immediately above, the primary outcome of prostate cancer-specific mortality is the recommended 'gold standard' for cancer screening trials, and the risk-reduction, conservatively estimated by intention-to-screen/effectiveness analysis (that included non-acceptors of the invitation to be screened) is at the lower bound—20% after an average of 2.1 screens per subject, over 9 years of follow-up—of effect-sizes usually found to be of interest to clinical and policy decision-makers regarding complex and expensive cancer screening programmes such as this one. [On the other hand, some widely implemented screening programmes, such as mammography in women 40–59 years old, appear to lead to rather small risk-reductions in cancer-site-specific mortality, closer to 15% (US Preventive Services Task Force2012b)]. Again, for men who were actually screened at least once, the efficacy effect-size was a more promising 27% reduction in the risk of prostate cancer death.

Question 9: Precision of primary outcome results

Suggested answer: The statistical precision, however, of the 20% (rate ratio) effectiveness estimate has a 95% confidence interval of 0.65–0.98, i.e. very close at the upper bound to the null hypothesis (rate ratio = 1.0, i.e. no effect at all). This indicates that the trial 'just barely' detected a statistically significant ($p = 0.04$) benefit of screening on the primary outcome, and that is slightly worrying. On the other hand, in sequentially analysed trials such as this one, there is an ethical onus to stop the trial when the pre-set 'boundary' for statistical significance (usually $p < 0.05$) is crossed during follow-up, so the authors cannot be blamed for reporting their outcomes at this point—to continue the trial would have raised other ethical issues. Nonetheless, the reporting of the considerable *adverse outcomes of PSA screening* detected in this trial lead one to reflect that the benefits are perhaps not as statistically soundly demonstrated as one would like.

The graph of the primary outcome against length of follow-up since randomization—figure 2 in Schroder et al. (2009) —is particularly convincing, since it shows just what would expect from a screening test that detects many slow-growing cases of cancer, and so is thought to provide a lead-time (vs the usual diagnosis after symptoms of cancer are felt) of '5–10 years'). Specifically, there is no detectable mortality effect (i.e. gap between the two curves of cumulative prostate cancer-mortality risk over time) until about 8 years after randomization (which was close in time to first offer of screening.)

Question 10: Other important outcomes all considered?
Suggested answer: Yes, those outcomes are well-reported, and they materially change one's view about the net risk–benefit balance of PSA screening—the striking aspect of this paper is that, more than for any other form of cancer screening already widely in place internationally, PSA screening has a high ratio of 'victims of screening' per beneficiary (see Question 3), due to both the relatively aggressive treatments frequently performed on men found to have early prostate cancer, and the very significant doubts that current science has about whether many of the very slow-growing, 'indolent' prostate cancers so-detected—especially in older men—would ever actually cause symptoms of any kind in that subject's remaining lifetime, before he is 'shuffled off the mortal coil' by another, competing cause of death. As noted above, this regrettable tendency of cancer screening is labelled 'length (-time)' or 'diagnostic' bias, and it leads to over-diagnosis and over-treatment of cancers (see 'Question 1' below). The abstract clearly cites the fact that, in this trial, some 48 additional ('i.e. beyond usual care frequency'—in the control group) men would have to be told they had prostate cancer, and offered either 'watch and wait' (for low-grade/stage tumours) or else definitive treatment (which is, at the current time, surgically, chemo-therapeutically, and/or radio-therapeutically aggressive), for each clear beneficiary (a subject whose death from prostate cancer was definitely delayed or prevented.) As pointed out, these 48 persons in the 'likely harmed' category, do not include many others who suffered psychological harm from the experience of having either:

1. A false-positive PSA test (some 76% of all 126,462 positive PSA tests in this study!) in that subsequent prostate needle biopsy, etc., found no cancer.

   Or

2. An 'over-diagnosed' cancer is detected—estimated to amount to up to half of the 4,235 screen-detected cancers in this trial—and they did not clearly benefit, in terms of the primary outcome, because that cancer was not a true threat to their health in their remaining lifetime.

As the accompanying *New England Journal of Medicine* editorial by Michael Barry (2009) argues, this risk–benefit profile is far worse than for, e.g. mammography screening for breast cancer, although increasingly there is a recognition that over-diagnosis of eventually-benign breast 'cancers' by mammography is a much larger problem than was thought to be the case during the first 30 years of official medical enthusiasm for mammography. Here are links to 2010 and 2011 lay-language summaries of this controversy, by the noted Canadian medical journalist Andre Picard:

1. http://www.theglobeandmail.com/life/health-and-fitness/routine-breast-scans-dont-affect-mortality/article572590/

2. http://m.theglobeandmail.com/life/health-and-fitness/health/condi-
tions/why-the-new-breast-cancer-screening-guidelines-make-sense/
article4179416/?service=mobile

Acknowledgments

Source: data from Schroder, F.H., et al., Screening and prostate-cancer mortality in a randomized European study, *New England Journal of Medicine*,
Volume 360, Number 13, pp. 1320–8, Copyright © 2009 Massachusetts
Medical Society. All rights reserved. Available from http://www.nejm.org/
doi/pdf/10.1056/NEJMoa0810084.

Chapter 8: Additional critical appraisal questions for RCTs of screening

**Question 1: If other health benefits of screening are claimed, e.g. screen-
detected cases with less advanced cancers, easier and cheaper to treat,
and with a better outcome, do the analyses adequately take account of
'length-(time) bias' and 'lead-time bias' to convince you that they are real
benefits, as opposed to, respectively, these two artefacts**

1. *'Length(-time)' or 'diagnostic' bias*: screening's inherent tendency to *preferentially* detect very slowly growing cancers, including some that would
not normally lead to symptoms in a patient's lifetime, leading in turn to
over-diagnosis and, potentially, *over-treatment*?

2. *Lead-time bias*: screening's misleading *apparent* capacity to add years
to the 'median/mean survival time after diagnosis,' and to increase the
'% 5 (or other *n*)-year survival after diagnosis,' even if cases detected by
screening die at the same average age as they would without screening?

Model answer: Yes, the paper clearly acknowledges the problems of 'length
(-time)'/'diagnostic' bias in PSA screening, and takes an appropriately conservative view regarding any claim that subjects, whose 'excess' prostate cancers were detected by screening, experienced net health benefits as a result.
Because of the strength of the RCT design, this study is able to precisely quantify the excess prostate cancer cases detected by the screening programme,
over the 9 years of follow-up, compared with those that were diagnosed in the
control 'usual care' group. Ignoring for a moment the differences in the total
number of subjects randomized to the two groups (72,890 screened versus
89,353 in the control group, within the predefined 'core' age-group—55–69 at
entry into the trial, presumably due to design peculiarities in some participating countries), there was an *excess* of 1,683 prostate cancers diagnosed in the
screened group (5,990 cancers: 8.2% of screened subjects) over the 9 years,
compared with the same-age control group (4,307 cancers: 4.8% of controls)

(figure 1 and table 1 in Schroder et al. (2009)). Critically, this design also shows that all the effort at diagnosing and treating these 1,683 extra cases only resulted in 102 fewer deaths due to prostate cancer during that same follow-up period (table 2, p. 1326 in Schroder et al. (2009)). Thus, we read the paper's final calculation, already cited, that 48 extra cancers had to be dealt with by both the patient, and his family and friends, and the health care system, for each death averted—probably the worst risk–benefit ratio ever conclusively demonstrated in a screening evaluation. There are other 'victims of inaccurate screening' as well though, which the paper does not emphasize, but for which the frequency in the trial can be calculated from the data presented.

Interestingly, no claims are made in this paper that some of the other men, whose cancers were detected at an 'early invasive stage,' may have benefited from having less aggressive therapy and perhaps better outcomes as well, as a result. That omission is probably related to the extremely poorly understood natural history of early prostate cancers, so that we really do not fully understand which ones will progress rapidly enough to become a health problem, in what is—for many older men, and most of those over 75—inevitably a rather short remaining lifetime in which to experience any benefit from screening, for a cancer that has (as the paper points out, p. 1326, bottom right in Schroder et al. (2009)) an estimated lead-time from PSA screening of '5–10 years.' Thus, we are told (p. 1327) that as many of 50% of the cancers detected by PSA screening represents full-fledged over-diagnoses.

Those of you previously trained in screening evaluation may have noted the absence, from this critical appraisal package, of the traditional '2 by 2' table of screening test validity, which is often used to summarize a screening test's sensitivity, specificity, and predictive values. This is no accident, and stems from the unusual situation here in this PSA screening trial, where one cannot readily compute 'sensitivity' for the test in the usual sense, since the test detected—after confirmatory testing by needle biopsy—more cancers than Mother Nature brought to light during follow-up in the control group, so that the 'sensitivity' is much more than '100%' (due to over-diagnosis, length and lead-time bias)—a nonsense notion! On the other hand, the positive predictive value of a positive PSA result is computed in table 1: about 24% overall. While this may seem high for a cancer screening test (it is!) its interpretation is fraught by the knowledge that the numerator—cancers detected—contains many over-diagnosed prostate-cancer cases (perhaps as many as 50% of the total). In summary, therefore, the usual '2 by 2' table of screening test validity is of limited utility in this situation.

Question 2: Are all the potential harms of screening identified and quantified—or at least acknowledged and discussed?

For example,

1. Additional anxiety and/or depression in those found to be screening-test positive, but who may have to wait weeks or months for the results

of confirmatory diagnostic testing (such as tissue biopsy), which are then negative?

2. Screening-induced side-effects of invasive confirmatory diagnostic testing—again, especially in those found to have either no disease as a result, or disease of such benign natural prognosis that its detection leads to over-diagnosis/over-treatment?

3. Screening-induced unnecessary side-effects of over-diagnosis and over-treatment, in this last group who are positive on confirmatory diagnostic testing, but whose disease is unlikely to have ever led to clinical consequences in their lifetimes, if left undetected by screening?

4. Screening-induced 'false reassurance' in persons who actually have prostate cancer, but are screened falsely as normal ('false negatives'), who then delay in presenting with symptoms of the undetected disease, later on, in the belief that their earlier negative screening test result was 100% accurate?

Model answer: Only the harms in categories 2 and 3 above are included in this paper's analyses—this is done partly by including all fatal side-effects/complications of both confirmatory needle biopsy (after positive PSA testing) and of subsequent prostate cancer treatment per se, as part of the primary outcome 'prostate cancer-specific mortality'. While this approach is not fully satisfactory, it is reasonable, given the formidable difficulties of ascertaining the full extent of *non-fatal* complications of invasive diagnostic testing and complex therapy, and of measuring—with repeated questionnaires to subjects with positive PSA results—the full psychological consequences of screening, especially for 'false' positives, whether they are among the 76% of positive PSA tests that did not have confirmatory diagnostic test (needle biopsy) results, or the potentially much more seriously affected group who were told they had prostate cancer after biopsy, but whose cases had up to a 50% probability of being an over-diagnosis). On the other hand, quantifying the 'false reassurance effect' is extremely difficult, since it requires detailed follow-up of screen-negative cases, and then some sort of complex assessment of any later-presenting cancer cases amongst those subjects, to determine if they may have presented later than otherwise would have been the case, due to false reassurance—a topic unlikely to be reported without bias by persons who typically believe they have had a 'true negative' test PSA result, given that the possibility of a false negative result is rarely communicated to the patient, by physicians ordering the test.

Question 3: Is the 'clinical efficiency' of the screening programme summarized in credible calculations of:

1) **'Number (of persons, over a given number of N years of follow-up) needed to screen' ('NNS') *per clear beneficiary?*** = the reciprocal of the

difference in the primary outcome rates in the unscreened and screened groups, after screening a specified number of times, over a specified number of years. It is particularly useful to calculate this as an intention-to-screen—or *effectiveness*—analysis, the number of persons who had to be *offered* the screen for each clear beneficiary, especially if the clinical encounter making this offer required significant resources—for example, to explain the potential benefits and risks of screening—and/or led to a relatively low rate of acceptance of screening. This is a non-valuated (non-economic) measure of screening programme efficiency, and is the first step in calculating its actual cost-effectiveness, but is much easier to compute (in that it required no cost assumptions) and to understand.

2. 'Number needed to harm' ('NNH')? = number of persons clearly adversely affected by screening (i.e. the sum of those experiencing any of the measured risks of screening already outlined) *per clear beneficiary*. This is a convenient summary of the risk-benefit balance of the screening programme, in that it quickly indicates if there are more 'victims' or more clear beneficiaries, overall.

Model answer: Yes—this paper is a model for screening RCT reporting, in that it not only calculates the NNT (1,410, after 2.1 screens on average, and 9 years of follow-up) and the NNH (48 extra men diagnosed with prostate cancer, and offered various treatments or 'watch and wait' per clear death averted, under the same conditions), both based conservatively on 'effectiveness'/intention-to-screen assumptions. As such, this rather definitive trial could be expected to put the final nails in the coffin of PSA screening. However, like many health policy 'zombies', it will probably turn out to have many lives—as the accompanying *New England Journal of Medicine* editorial by Barry (2009) implies. This is partly because it is rather difficult to explain to the lay public all of the above and, in particular, how screening can cause net harm. As well, there is the screening 'popularity paradox', cited by Raffle and Gray (2007, p. 68): 'The greater the harm through over diagnosis and overtreatment from screening, the more screened people there are who *believe* they owe their health, or even their life, to the programme.'

Acknowledgements

Source: data from Angela E. Raffle and J. A. Muir Gray, *Screening: Evidence and Practice*, Oxford University Press, Oxford, UK, © 2007 Oxford University Press.

Notes

Chapter 2

1. Lest the reader infer that the authors are 'too negative' about prevention, we would point to a well-established and widely cited literature that provides detailed examples of successful medical and public health interventions which are largely preventive in nature, epitomized by the classic ten-part series 'Ten great public health achievements' produced some years ago by the U.S. national public health agency (Centers for Disease and Prevention 1999). Similar arguments have been made many times since (e.g. Centers for Disease and Prevention 2011), so the authors have chosen not to repeat them in this book.

Chapter 3

2. As we shall see in Chapter 10, the prescient investigations of Graunt and Farr established the field of 'social' epidemiology, which has flowered since the 1980s, particularly in the UK. Those hundreds of studies, carried out in many diverse cultural and geographic settings, have 'clearly demonstrated that most diseases and causes of death are not only more common in the poor, but actually more common in the middle classes than in the privileged—creating what is known as 'social gradients' in health (European Commission 2013; Marmot 2010; Marmot et al. 2008; Wilkinson and Marmot 2003).

3. Cholera is an acute infectious disease caused by a bacterium, characterized by severe diarrhoea and vomiting, leading to dehydration and death without urgent medical treatment.

4. For those wishing to learn more about John Snow's investigations 'On the mode of communication of Cholera' can be read here: http://www.ph.ucla.edu/epi/snow/snowbook2.html (accessed 27th July 2015) and the book by Vinten-Johansen et al. (2003) as well as the John Snow Society (http://www.johnsnowsociety.org/ (accessed 27th July 2015) would be good places to start.

5. One is struck by the parallel here with the experience of Joseph Goldberger in the USA some decades later. Goldberger also had to fight mainstream medical thinking for many years before pellagra was widely accepted as deriving from a nutritional deficiency, rather than an infection. He also had to indulge—much like Pettenkofer—in experiments wherein he deliberately tried to infect himself, and his friends and relatives with the bodily fluids and belongings of pellagra victims; since those efforts were unsuccessful, they went a long way towards disproving that pellagra was an infectious disease. It seems that epidemiology was rather a hazardous profession in that era.

6. Subsequent research suggests, however, that the credit given to Snow for the beneficial effects of removing the pump handle, may have been over-stated; careful examination of the graph of daily new cases near Broad Street reveals that the outbreak was already beginning the decline phase typical of a 'point-source' epidemic of disease caused by temporarily contaminated water or food (McLeod 2000). Ironically, epidemiologists now have a term for situations where a disease declines in frequency about the time that a health intervention is locally implemented, but subsequent investigations reveal that the latter may well not have caused the former. This is called 'riding the pump-handle down.' The implication, of course, is that public health authorities should not take credit for what may well have occurred anyway.

7. The definition and uses of these terms are covered in all basic epidemiology texts—for example, Young (1998)—which assumes no prior relevant knowledge, and deftly avoids statistically complex explanations.

Chapter 4

8. Sometimes referred to as 'primary studies'

9. Evidence for Policy and Practice Information and Co-ordinating Centre (EPPI-Centre): http://eppi.ioe.ac.uk/cms/

Chapter 5

10. In epidemiological terms, persons with a Body Mass Index (BMI) between 25 and 30 are 'overweight;' those with a BMI over 30 are 'obese' and those under 25 are normal or, if under 20 'underweight' (Butland et al. 2007). Serious health effects from overweight begin at BMIs just under 30, increasing as BMI increases, with very high risks indeed for those whose BMI is over 35 to 40 (Butland et al. 2007).

11. There are many other, more invasive and intensive treatments for full-blown obesity, which are justified when the condition is severe enough to cause an imminent threat to health, e.g. drugs and various surgical interventions. Our focus here, however, is on the prevention of overweight in normal persons, and of obesity among overweight persons, in keeping with the theme of this book.

Chapter 6

12. For example, the one of the authors (JF) lived in a small town in Tanzania in the 1970s, when many local people, still eking out a living as subsistence farmers, ate a traditional diet consisting of a large cup of milky, sugar-sweetened tea ('chai' in Swahili) in the morning, followed by one other large meal in the afternoon, the centrepiece of which was a heaping, shared bowl of maize-meal porridge the approximate consistency of wallpaper paste ('ugali'), accompanied by whatever flavourful sauce ('mchuzi') could be scrounged, usually made of beans, with perhaps a tomato and onion per cooking pot—with meat and fowl reserved for special ceremonial and celebratory occasions. There was little likelihood that reporting on such a diet would be prone to error, given the diet's extraordinary monotony.

13. Other dietary sources of omega-3s exist, such as linseed, also known as flaxseed, which is the usual source of these nutrients fed specially to laying chickens, so that their eggs can be marketed as high in omega-3 fatty acids. However, until the modern omega-3 enrichment of eggs and other foods for the health-conscious consumer, very few persons in the developed world routinely ate significant amounts of flaxseed or its oil.

14. 'Confounding' is defined as 'Loosely, the distortion of a measure of the effect of an exposure on an outcome due to the association of the exposure with other factors that influence the occurrence of the outcome. Confounding occurs when all or part of the apparent association between the exposure and the outcome is in fact accounted for by other variables that affect the outcome and are not themselves affected by exposure' (p.55, Porta 2008).

    Text extracts from Porta, M.S (Ed.), *A Dictionary of Epidemiology, Sixth Edition*, Oxford University Press, New York, USA, Copyright © International Epidemiological Association, Inc., 2014, reproduced by permission of Oxford University Press USA.

15. This very pro-walnut coverage of the study may well have been aided and abetted by one of the co-authors' funders, the California Walnut Commission, who are clearly named in the paper as having provided the investigators with an 'unrestricted educational grant' and therefore—and this is entirely credible—had no influence over the actual study design and analysis. The difficulty is that even the best investigators have no control over how some parties disseminate their results.

16. Notably, a team (Bao et al. 2013) analysing this same NHS dataset, as well as a large cohort of American male health care professionals, published—about the same time as Pan et al. (2013)—a very sophisticated analysis showing that the consumption of any kind of nuts (either from trees, or peanuts) at the dose of seven or more occasions per week, conferred a 20% reduction in the risk of death from all causes, which was not much reduced by adjustment for an equally large number of potential confounders. However, that study had insufficient numbers of deaths due to diabetes, to address the research question addressed by Pan et al. (2013).

17. Just as Churchill famously said about democracy, one could also say about peer-review, that 'Indeed, it has been said that democracy is the worst form of Government except all those other forms that have been tried from time to time' (from a House of Commons speech on Nov. 11, Hansard, 1947).

    Reproduced from Parliament Bill, HC Deb 11 November 1947 vol 444 cc203–321, under the Open Parliament Licence v3.0, available from http://hansard. millbanksystems.com/commons/1947/nov/11/parliament-bill

Chapter 7

18. Hygeia was the ancient Greek goddess of health, cleanliness and sanitation; from her name has come this lovely word, now consigned to the rather narrow

meaning of 'related to sanitation or cleanliness.' However, just over a century ago, the word had a much broader connotation, related to the preservation of health in general, by any of a wide range of behaviours and habits that protect from disease and death (Oxford English Dictionary 2015).

19. Examples include eating cycad seeds (or fruit bats that have eaten these seeds) and developing a severe neurodegenerative disease, previously endemic on the Pacific island of Guam (Lytico-bodig disease (Sacks 1997)); consuming a particular lentil widely eaten in South Asia in the past, especially in times of famine, that leads to nerve damage (lathryism (Spencer et al. 1993)); and many parasitic diseases caused by consuming contaminated meat, fish or produce, especially if eaten raw (any tropical medicine text describes dozens of these).

20. The quality-adjusted life-year (QALY) is a measure of disease burden, including both the quality and the quantity of life lived. It is used in assessing the value for money of a medical intervention (Appleby et al. 2007).

21. The notion that health benefits, and risks, of any preventive treatment, are not as 'important' if they occur far into the future as they are if they occur much closer in time, is formally acknowledged and quantified in a health-economic calculation called 'discounting' or 'time-preference.' As we shall see later in this chapter, health economic studies that meet standard quality criteria always include a range of percentage-per-year-in-the-future rates for discounting the value of all future events, as well as costs, to quantify the fact that a 'bird in the hand (now) is always worth more than a bird in the bush (in the future)'. Later in this chapter the authors discuss the effect of such discount rates on the cost-effectiveness of statins.

22. Readers interested in calculating their own risk of cardiovascular disease (CVD) or death in the next decade should be aware that some of the 'cardiovascular risk-calculators' in wide use are not well validated against cohort studies that have measured all the relevant risk factors at baseline, and then counted all important instances of CVD over many years of follow-up. A recent, well-done validation study by Collins and Altman (2012) showed that, of the risk-calculators in wide use in the UK, the QRISK2 calculator is the best, in terms of accurately predicting risk. It is available at: http://www.qrisk.org/index.php. Before logging on to use it for yourself, you will need to know your basic medical history, your current systolic blood pressure, as well as your total and HDL cholesterol levels (and the ratio of the former to the latter), and—to make the most use of its sophisticated allowance for social class (lower social class is a major contributor to CVD in the UK and most developed-country settings, as the authors will discuss in Chapter 10)—your postcode of residence in the UK.

23. On the other hand, those questioning the new NICE guidance of 2014 point to the fact that 'Atorvastatin has never been demonstrated to reduce mortality for primary prevention [in] any clinical study' (Thompson et al. 2014, p.1).

24. If such low compliance rates are indeed generalizable, published tallies of projected benefits would have to be pro-rated accordingly. The NICE 2014 cost-effectiveness study cited in Table 7.1 explicitly modelled the effects of non-compliance with statins as part of their 'sensitivity analysis,' and found

that the overall ICERs did not change much. This is because those who stop taking a daily drug stop both the related expenses entailed in their care, and also reduce their future health benefits to zero, at least eventually. However, this rather technocratic calculation does not acknowledge the fact that substantially reduced long-term compliance with indefinite daily drug treatments, especially for asymptomatic conditions (as is common in primary preventive statin therapy), carries with it a proportionate reduction in the overall impact on the overall mortality and morbidity burden of cardiovascular disease, at the population level, of such individually-based prevention strategies. Moreover, there is substantial evidence that such individually-based preventive strategies typically achieve much higher levels of initial uptake, and ongoing compliance, in higher socioeconomic groups, thus potentially widening already steep socioeconomic health inequalities for cardiovascular outcomes (Capewell and Graham 2010).

Chapter 8

25. This effort was arguably all in vain, in that two of these three types of under-evaluated screening—breast and testicular self-examination—for which there was then no solid proof of effectiveness—continued to be widely promoted and taken up in most developed countries for some decades. Notably, however, the tide has now turned against Breast Self-Examination to detect breast cancer (US Preventive Services Task Force, 2009b). We now have, but did not have in the 1980s, convincing RCTs of stool-for-occult-blood testing's effectiveness for reducing colorectal cancer deaths (US Preventive Services Task Force, 2008); the 1985 papers cited above (Frank 1985a,b,c) critically analysed that screening test and strongly urged it not be routinely used on patients at normal risk of colorectal cancer until those RCTs reported. That advice was pretty much ignored.

26. This is especially true for cancers, because of screening tests' tendency to over-diagnose mild cases that would do well anyway, and also their typically high 'false-positive rate'. The false-positive rate is the proportion of positive screening results that are not subsequently found to actually have cancer after full, and typically invasive, investigation. In the case of prostate cancer, this investigation of men with positive PSA tests normally consists of radiologically-guided needle biopsy of the prostate through the rectal wall; this biopsy carries a small but definite risk of haemorrhage or infection complications. Scans, x-rays and other studies may also be required to rule out cancer spread to other organs. In the trial by Schröder et al. (2009), only 24% of the 20,437 positive PSA tests in patients who underwent this invasive confirmatory investigation turned out to have detectable cancers in their prostate. And that is an over-estimate of the clinically-meaningful cancers that would have likely caused symptoms or death in their lifetimes, due to over-diagnosis. Estimates of the proportion of PSA-detected cancers that are over-diagnosed range from 50% to 70% (Barry, 2009; Miller, 2012; Schröder et al., 2012). If that is true, then only 8% to 12% [i.e. 24% X (1-(0.5 to 0.7))] of the positive PSA tests in the ERSPC trial were due to clinically meaningful cancers which were truly threatening the patient's health. The rest of the PSA positives were 'artefacts of screening'.

27. Uncritical promotion of screening is usually led by specialist physicians who have become understandably disheartened by years of seeing patients who have late-stage disease by the time they present for care with symptoms—and who therefore do badly. While their intent is laudable, one of the authors (JF) found that it to be virtually impossible to counter the views of these senior clinicians with epidemiological reasoning. This led to his abandoning field of screening research after 1991; it was discouraging to argue against poorly-validated screening practices, at that point in North American medical history. In Canada, despite the need to make efficient use of public monies in its well-established publicly-funded healthcare system, the strong American cultural belief that 'more testing is always better' had already taken a firm hold in the minds of the public and professionals alike.

28. The 2012 publication of data from two further years of follow-up of all ESPRC subjects for further cancer cases and deaths—but without any further screening being done—found a slightly more favourable NNS of 1,055 men (936 for all follow-up data, beyond 12 years) needing to be invited for screening to extend one life (Schröder et al., 2012). This is not unexpected, since the cumulative death rates from prostate cancer only began to diverge after about 7 years of follow-up from randomisation, and continued to diverge as long as follow-up occurred. This reflects the expected lengthy 'lead time' between finding a potentially lethal prostate tumour by screening, and the actual death of the patient from it had it not been detected and treated, because most prostate cancers grow very slowly. Notably, however, the extra two-years of follow-up did not substantially change the rate of occurrence of harms from screening and its consequences, so that the NNH remained similarly high in the 2012 publication, at 37 (33 for all follow-up data, beyond 12 years) men who had to be diagnosed with cancer, and offered treatment, for each man whose life was extended by screening, reported in the 2012 publication—slightly more favourable than the NNH of 48. Again, this was to be expected, since the actual screening had stopped by the last few years of follow-up, and it is the screening and treatment for the cases it detects, that causes the harmful side-effects—usually rather rapidly.

29. The authors have then greatly simplified the actual mathematical modelling required, because we could not find a published model's results which are precisely comparable to the published models summarized about, for the effects of a recommended 'lifetime' of mammography (biennially, age 50-69). The authors have assumed that: 1) that the benefits of screening, in terms of lives extended per thousand persons screened, are proportionate to the number of times PSA testing is done—this is rather dubious, in part because initial screens typically have higher yields of cancer than subsequent screens, but it gives the benefit of the doubt to PSA screening; 2) the various harms of PSA screening, per thousand men screened, are also approximately proportional to the number of times they are screened; this is quite credible, in that most of the harms occur early on in follow-up after each screen, in the form of false positive PSA tests which are negative on prostate biopsy; the anxiety and complications of biopsy, and the treatment side-effects for men found to have cancer and treated, of whom at least 50% are estimated to be victims of 'over-diagnosis'.

30. One promising option, for all types of patient education about any preventive intervention, is high-quality and scientifically reliable web-based videos, such as those of Dr Mike Evans at the University of Toronto. At the time of writing he has just released a superb whiteboard talk about PSA testing (https://www.youtube.com/watch?v=bTgS0DuhaUU).

31. This term means that the patient is closely monitored clinically and often by repeat laboratory tests, for any evidence of cancer progression, but is not treated for the cancer itself. Guidelines are available on what criteria, based on both clinical and biopsy considerations, should be used to select patients for this conservative management approach, but they are still controversial (US Preventive Services Task Force, 2012b).

Chapter 9

32. The reader may, at this point, counter that considerable fanfare has heralded the discovery of single gene defects that greatly increase the risk of common and severe later-life diseases, such as the genetic variants *BRCA1* and *BRCA2*. It is true that these genes massively increase the risk of developing breast cancer over a lifetime; however, they are too rare in the general population to account for more than a tiny fraction of the annual breast cancers in any developed country. (More inbred ethnic groups, on the other hand, can have much higher frequencies of these genes.) Thus, *BRCA1* only occurs in 0.1–0.2% of North American women, so causing less than 5% of breast cancers in the general population. As a result, something like 2,500 healthy women would have to be screened (the Number Needed to Screen: NNS—Chapter 8) in order to prevent one case of cancer in the general population (Vineis et al. 2001). Such testing may well be worthwhile, however, in a high-risk family or ethnic group that has a much higher frequency of *BRCA1*. This point will be revisited later in this chapter, with respect to screening for the future risk of colorectal cancer using currently available, but generally rather uncommon, genetic markers.

33. Lest it be thought that the apparently much simpler causation of single-gene disorders has led to successful interventions to prevent them from developing, through, for example, simple testing of populations at high risk, followed by genetic counselling, it is instructive to look at the example of cystic fibrosis (CF). Despite decades of earnest and skilled research since the initial identification of the location of that disorder's defective gene in 1989, there is still no easy way to eliminate the disease, because it turns out that there are hundreds of different variants (versions) of the 'CF gene', carrying varying degrees of risk, for varying severities and natural histories of CF. In other words, the prevention of even single gene disorders can be much more complicated than one might expect (Nussbaum et al. 2001, p. 222–5).

34. The two-by-two table was, rather ironically in retrospect, used in a series of papers in the mid-1980s by one of the authors (JF) to analyse the risks and benefits of stool-for-occult-blood (SOB) screening for CRC, before several

large randomized control trials of that screening test had reported on their results (Frank 1985a,b,c). This three-part series of articles was written as a warning against premature adoption of that cancer screening test, at a time when many primary care physicians in North America were already routinely using the SOB test on all their patients past mid-life. This practice was, at the time, widespread in medical practice in spite of the fact that there was then no evidence at all that the test led to more benefits than risks. It was thus a situation remarkably prescient of the giant, decades-long wave of un-validated PSA screening for prostate cancer which began in North America a few years later (Chapter 8). However, unlike PSA screening, SOB screening is still recommended by respected authorities (US Preventive Services Task Force 2008). It has the problem, however, that it is so much less sensitive and specific than the gold-standard—screening colonoscopy—that only the very high cost (and limited availability of endoscopists) argues for its continued use. Indeed, at least one physician-researcher has tellingly written that virtually all informed physicians do not bother with SOB screening. Physicians just request screening endoscopy about every decade after they turn 50 (Detsky 2001).

35. As explained in Chapter 5.

Chapter 10

36. Note that these ten rank-ordered deciles of socioeconomic status utilized in the Scottish annual reports on health inequalities are based on the postcode of residence of all citizens in the entire population—clustered into 6,505 'data-zones' for about 5 million Scots, so that the resultant geographical areas are very small indeed. Furthermore, these zones' boundaries are set so as to respect natural communities within which social class is likely to be more homogeneous, such as public housing estates—rather than 'gerrymandering' across diverse communities, which tends to understate inequalities as a whole.

37. This corollary is directly analogous to what Geoffrey Rose (Chapter 5) pointed out for the population burden of illness attributable to most chronic disease risk factors: most diseases cases (e.g. cardiovascular disease) due to any given risk factor which has more than one level of possible exposure arise in the middle of the bell-curve that describes the population distribution of the risk factor—e.g. serum cholesterol, as we saw in Chapter 7.

38. This situation has largely changed nowadays, in that most TB in developed countries arises from a combination of reactivated old cases in elderly persons who first became infected many decades ago, when the condition was ubiquitous, and cases amongst immigrants who have left poorer countries where most individuals are still infected in childhood (as was true in Europe only a century ago). Even a small TB re-activation rate in later life, amongst immigrants, dwarfs the risk in European non-immigrants, apart from the oldest old. In North America and Australia, this pattern is further complicated by the continuing (though

much reduced) epidemic of TB among aboriginal peoples, who appear to have been especially susceptible to the disease, after they first encountered it when it arrived with white colonialists (Comstock 2007).

39. By 'relative' inequalities, the authors mean the relative risk of adverse outcomes between SES groups, as opposed 'absolute' inequalities, which is the difference in risk, a distinction introduced in Chapter 3. Since most common diseases' incidence and mortality rates have steadily come down in developed countries in recent decades (obesity and its complications, such as Type II diabetes, excepted), one would expect absolute inequalities to have come down spontaneously as all social classes benefit to at least some degree from improved living conditions and medical advances. Therefore relative inequalities are considered a more stringent test of whether inequality reduction has occurred. Recent comprehensive studies by Mackenbach et al. (2015) show that in fact most EU mortality inequalities by SES have been remarkably stable over the last few decades, with a few absolute inequalities declining, but almost all relative inequalities stable or increasing.

References

Abramson, J.D., Rosenberg, H.G., Jewell, N., and Wright, J.M. (2013). Should people at low risk of cardiovascular disease take a statin? *British Medical Journal*, 347, f6123.

Akhtar, P.C., Currie, D.B., Currie, C.E., and Haw, S.J. (2007). Changes in child exposure to environmental tobacco smoke (CHETS) study after implementation of smoke-free legislation in Scotland. *British Medical Journal*, 335, 545.

Alpha-Tocopherol Beta Carotene Cancer Prevention Study Group (1994). The effect of vitamin E and beta carotene on the incidence of lung cancer and other cancers in male smokers. *New England Journal of Medicine*, 330, 1029–35.

Anderson, G.L., Limacher, M., Assaf, A.R., et al. (2004). Effects of conjugated equine estrogen in postmenopausal women with hysterectomy: the Women's Health Initiative randomized controlled trial. *Journal of the American Medical Association*, 291, 1701–12.

Anderson, G.M., Bronskill, S.E., Mustard, C.A., Culyer, A., Alter, D.A., and Manuel, D.G. (2005). Both clinical epidemiology and population health perspectives can define the role of health care in reducing health disparities. *Journal of Clinical Epidemiology*, 58, 757–62.

Appleby, J., Devlin, N., and Parkin, D. (2007). NICE's cost effectiveness threshold. *British Medical Journal*, 335, 358–9.

Armitage, J., Baigent, C., and Collins, R. (2014). Misrepresentation of statin safety evidence. *Lancet*, 384, 1263–4.

Bao, Y., Han, J., Hu, F.B., et al. (2013). Association of nut consumption with total and cause-specific mortality. *New England Journal of Medicine*, 369, 2001–11.

Barry, M.J. (2009). Screening for prostate cancer–the controversy that refuses to die. *New England Journal of Medicine*, 360, 1351–4.

Beasley, R.P., Hwang, L.Y., Lin, C.C., and Chien, C.S. (1981). Hepatocellular carcinoma and hepatitis B virus. A prospective study of 22 707 men in Taiwan. *Lancet*, 2, 1129–33.

Bekelman, J.E., Li, Y., and Gross, C.P. (2003). Scope and impact of financial conflicts of interest in biomedical research: a systematic review. *Journal of the American Medical Association*, 289, 454–65.

Bhattacharya, S. (2005). Up to 140,000 heart attacks linked to Vioxx. *New Scientist*, London. Available at: http://www.newscientist.com/article/dn6918-up-to-140000-heart-attacks-linked-to-vioxx.html#.VUd1BGO4JoV (accessed 18 August 2015).

Boffetta, P., Couto, E., Wichmann, J., et al. (2010). Fruit and vegetable intake and overall cancer risk in the European Prospective Investigation into Cancer and Nutrition (EPIC). *Journal of the National Cancer Institute*, 102, 529–37.

Bollet, A.J. (1992). Politics and pellagra: the epidemic of pellagra in the U.S. in the early twentieth century. *Yale Journal of Biology and Medicine*, **65**, 211–21.

Boseley, S. (2014). NHS medicines watchdog lowers bar for statins prescriptions [18 July 2014]. *The Guardian*, London. Available at: http://www.theguardian. com/society/2014/jul/18/nhs-medicines-watchdog-nice-statins-guideline (accessed 18 August 2015).

Bresalier, R.S., Sandler, R.S., Quan, H., et al. (2005). Cardiovascular events associated with rofecoxib in a colorectal adenoma chemoprevention trial. *New England Journal of Medicine*, **352**, 1092–102.

Brownell, K.D. and **Warner, K.E.** (2009). The perils of ignoring history: big tobacco played dirty and millions died. how similar is big food? *Milbank Quarterly*, **87**, 259–94.

Buck, C., Llopis, A., Nájera, E., and **Terris, M.** (1988). *The challenge of epidemiology: issues and selected readings*. Pan American Health Organization, Washington, DC.

Butland, B., Jebb, S., Kopelman, P., et al. (2007). *Tackling obesities: future choices— project report*, 2nd edn. Department of Innovation, Universities and Skills, London.

Cain, D.M., Loewenstein, G., and **Moore, D.A.** (2005). The dirt on coming clean: perverse effects of disclosing conflicts of interest. *Journal of Legal Studies*, **34**, 1–25.

Campbell, T.C. and **Campbell, T.M., II** (2005). *The China study: the most comprehensive study of nutrition ever conducted and the startling implications for diet, weight loss and long-term health*. Benbella, Dallas, Tx.

Canadian Task Force on Preventive Health Care (not dated). *Canadian Task Force on Preventive Healthcare*. University of Calgary, Calgary, Alberta. Available at: http:// canadiantaskforce.ca/ (accessed 18 August 2015).

Capewell, S. (2014). Presentation to the European Public Health Association Conference in Glasgow on 21 November 2014. Available at: www.eupha.org (accessed 18 August 2015).

Capewell, S. and **Graham, H.** (2010). Will cardiovascular disease prevention widen health inequalities? *PLoS Medicine*, **7**, e1000320.

Carter, A.A., Gomes, T., Camacho, X., Juurlink, D.N., Shah, B.R., and **Mamdani, M.M.** (2013). Risk of incident diabetes among patients treated with statins: population based study. *British Medical Journal*, **346**, f2610.

Catalano, R. and **Frank, J.** (2001). Detecting the effect of medical care on mortality. *Journal of Clinical Epidemiology*, **54**, 830–6.

Centers for Disease Prevention (CDC) (1999). Ten great public health achievements— United States, 1900–1999. *MMWR Morbidity and Mortality Weekly Reports*, **48**, 241–3.

Centers for Disease Prevention (CDC) (2011). Ten great public health achievements— worldwide, 2001–2010. *MMWR Morbidity and Mortality Weekly Reports*, **60**, 814–18.

Centre for Reviews and Dissemination (2015). University of York, Centre for Reviews and Dissemination. University of York, York. Available at: http://www.crd.york. ac.uk/CRDWeb/HomePage.asp (accessed 18 August 2015).

Chen, C-L., Tetri, L.H., Neuschwander-Tetri, B.A., Huang, S.S., and Huang, J.S. (2011). A mechanism by which dietary trans fats cause atherosclerosis. *Journal of Nutritional Biochemistry*, 22, 649–55.

Choi, B.C., Hunter, D.J., Tsou, W., and Sainsbury, P. (2005). Diseases of comfort: primary cause of death in the 22nd century. *Journal of Epidemiology Community Health*, 59, 1030–4.

Cholesterol Treatment Trialists' Collaborators, Mihaylova, B., Emberson, J., et al. (2012). The effects of lowering LDL cholesterol with statin therapy in people at low risk of vascular disease: meta-analysis of individual data from 27 randomised trials. *Lancet*, 380, 581–90.

Chou, R., Croswell, J.M., Dana, T., et al. (2011). Screening for prostate cancer: a review of the evidence for the US Preventive Services Task Force. *Annals of Internal Medicine*, 155, 762–71.

Chowdhury, S., Dent, T., Pashayan, N., et al. (2013). Incorporating genomics into breast and prostate cancer screening: assessing the implications. *Genetics in Medicine*, 15, 423–32.

Clasen, T.F., Alexander, T.K. Sinckair, D., Boisson, S., Peletz, R., Chang, H.H., Majorin, F., and Cairncross, S. (2015). Interventions to improve water quality for preventing diarrhoea. *Cochrane Database of Systematic Reviews*, Issue 10. Art. No.: CD004794.

Collins, G.S. and Altman, D.G. (2012). Predicting the 10 year risk of cardiovascular disease in the United Kingdom: independent and external validation of an updated version of QRISK2. *British Medical Journal*, 344, e4181.

Comstock, G.W. (2007). Tuberculosis. In: Holland, W.W., Olsen, J., Florey, and C.d.V. (eds), *The development of modern epidemiology: personal reports from those who were there*, pp.147–55. Oxford University Press, Oxford.

Craig, P., Cooper, C., Gunnell, D., et al. (2011). Using natural experiments to evaluate population health interventions: guidance for producers and users of evidence. Medical Research Council, London. Available at: http://www.mrc.ac.uk/documents/ pdf/natural-experiments-guidance/ (accessed 18 August 2015).

Craig, P., Dieppe, P., Macintyre, S., Michie, S., Nazareth, I., and Petticrew, M. (2008). Developing and evaluating complex interventions: the new Medical Research Council guidance. *British Medical Journal*, 337, e1655.

Crowcroft, N.S., Hamid, J.S., Deeks, S.L., and Frank, J. (2012). Human papilloma virus vaccination programs reduce health inequity in most scenarios: a simulation study. *BMC Public Health*, 12, 935.

Culver, A.L., Ockene, I.S., Balasubramanian, R., et al. (2012). Statin use and risk of diabetes mellitus in postmenopausal women in the Women's Health Initiative. *Archives of Internal Medicine*, 172, 144–52.

Culyer, A.J. (2005). *The dictionary of health economics*. Edward Elgar, Cheltenham.

Dahlgren, G. and Whitehead, M. (2007). Policies and strategies to promote social equity in health. Institute for Future Studies, Stockholm. Available at: http://www.iffs.se/en/publication/policies-and-strategies-to-promote-social-equity-in-health/ (accessed 18 August 2015).

Des Jarlais, D.C., Lyles, C., Crepaz, N., and the TREND Group, (2004). Improving the reporting quality of nonrandomized evaluations of behavioral and public health interventions: the TREND statement. *American Journal of Public Health*, **94**, 361–6.

Detsky, A.S. (2001). Screening for colon cancer—can we afford colonoscopy? *New England Journal of Medicine*, **345**, 607–8.

Diao, D., Wright, J.M., Cundiff, D.K., and Gueyffier, F. (2012). Pharmacotherapy for mild hypertension. *Cochrane Database of Systematic Reviews*, Issue 8, Art. No.: CD006742.

Doerr, M. and Eng, C. (2012). Personalised care and the genome. *British Medical Journal*, **344**, e3174.

Doll, R. and Hill, A.B. (1950). Smoking and carcinoma of the lung; preliminary report. *British Medical Journal*, **2**, 739–48.

Doll, R. and Hill, A.B. (1964a). Mortality in relation to smoking: ten years' observations of British doctors. *British Medical Journal*, **1**, 1460–7.

Doll, R. and Hill, A.B. (1964b). Mortality in relation to smoking: ten years' observations of British doctors. *British Medical Journal*, **1**, 1399–410.

Dormuth, C.R., Filion, K.B., Paterson, J.M., et al. (2014). Higher potency statins and the risk of new diabetes: multicentre, observational study of administrative databases. *British Medical Journal*, **348**, g3244.

Doyle, J. and the Cochrane Public Health Group (2009). About The Cochrane Collaboration (Cochrane Review Groups (CRGs)). Issue 12, Art. No.: PUBHLTH. Available at: http://onlinelibrary.wiley.com/o/cochrane/clabout/articles/PUBHLTH/frame.html (accessed 18 August 2015).

Drummond, M.F. (1997). *Methods for the economic evaluation of health care programmes*, 2nd edn. Oxford University Press, Oxford.

Ebrahim, S. and Casas, J.P. (2012). Statins for all by the age of 50 years? *Lancet* **380**, 545–7.

Estruch, R., Ros, E., Salas-Salvado, J., et al. (2013). Primary prevention of cardiovascular disease with a Mediterranean diet. *New England Journal of Medicine*, **368**:1279–90.

European Commission (2013). Health inequalities in the EU—final report of a consortium. Sir Michael Marmot, Consortium lead. Available at: http://www.hfcm.eu/web/catalog/item/553-health-inequalities-in-the-eu-final-report-of-a-consortium-consortium-lead-sir-michael-marmot (accessed 13 December 2015).

Evans, R.G., Barer, M.L., and Marmor, T.R. (1994). *Why are some people healthy and others not?: the determinants of health of populations*. A. de Gruyter, New York, NY.

Everett, T., Bryant, A., Griffin, M.F., Martin-Hirsch, P.P., Forbes, C.A., and Jepson, R.G. (2011). Interventions targeted at women to encourage the uptake of cervical screening. *Cochrane Database of Systematic Reviews* Issue 5, Art. No.: CD002834.

Finckenauer, J.O. (1982). *Scared straight and the panacea phenomenon.* Prentice-Hall, Englewood Cliffs, NJ.

Finucane, M.M., Stevens, G.A., Cowan, M.J., et al., (2011). National, regional, and global trends in body-mass index since 1980: systematic analysis of health examination surveys and epidemiological studies with 960 country-years and 9.1 million participants. *Lancet,* **337,** 557–67.

Frank, J. (1985a). Occult-blood screening for colorectal carcinoma: the benefits. *American Journal of Preventive Medicine,* **1,** 3–9.

Frank, J. (1985b). Occult-blood screening for colorectal carcinoma: the risks. *American Journal of Preventive Medicine,* **1,** 25–32.

Frank, J. (1985c). Occult-blood screening for colorectal carcinoma: the yield and the costs. *American Journal of Preventive Medicine,* **1,** 18–24.

Frank, J., Bromley, C., Doi, L., et al. (2015). Seven key investments for health equity across the lifecourse: Scotland versus the rest of the UK. *Social Science and Medicine,* **140,** 136–46.

Frank, J., Di Ruggiero, E., McInnes, R.R., Kramer, M., and Gagnon, F. (2006a). Large life-course cohorts for characterizing genetic and environmental contributions: the need for more thoughtful designs. *Epidemiology,* **17,** 595–8.

Frank, J., Lomax, G., Baird, P., and Lock, M. (2006b). Interactive role of genes and the environment. In: Heymann, J., Hertzman, C., Barer, M.L., and Evans, R.G. (eds.) *Healthier societies: from analysis to action,* pp. 11–34. Oxford University Press, Oxford.

Frank, J. and Mai, V. (1985). Breast self-examination in young women: more harm than good? *Lancet,* **2,** 654–7.

Garbe, C. and Leiter, U. (2009). Melanoma epidemiology and trends. *Clinical Dermatology,* **27,** 3–9.

Gee, D. (2008). Establishing evidence for early action: the prevention of reproductive and developmental harm. *Basic & Clinical Pharmacology & Toxicology,* **102,** 257–66.

Glantz, S.A. (1996). *The cigarette papers.* University of California Press, Berkeley.

Godlee, F. (2013). Statins for all over 50? No. *British Medical Journal,* **347,** f6412.

Godlee, F. (2014a). Adverse effects of statins. *British Medical Journal,* **348,** g3306.

Godlee, F. (2014b). Statins and the BMJ. *British Medical Journal,* **349,** g5038.

Goldacre, B. (2014). Statins are a mess: we need better data, and shared decision making. *British Medical Journal,* **348,** g3306.

Goldacre, B., Godlee, F., Heneghan, C., et al. (2014). Open letter: European Medicines Agency should remove barriers to access clinical trial data. *British Medical Journal,* **348,** g3768.

Goldberg, E.M. and Morrison, S.L. (1963). Schizophrenia and social class. *British Journal of Psychiatry*, **109**, 785–802.

Goldstein, D.B. (2009). Common genetic variation and human traits. *New England Journal of Medicine*, **360**, 1696–8.

Graunt, J.F.R.S. (1662). *Natural and political observations mentioned in a following Index, and made upon the Bills of Mortality ... With reference to the government, religion, trade, growth, ayre, and diseases of the said city*. London.

Greenwald, P. (2003). β-Carotene and lung cancer: a lesson for future chemoprevention investigations? *Journal of the National Cancer Institute*, **95**, E1.

Greving, J.P., Visseren, F.L., de Wit, G.A., and Algra, A. (2011). Statin treatment for primary prevention of vascular disease: whom to treat? Cost-effectiveness analysis. *British Medical Journal*, **342**, d1672.

Gueyffier, F. and Wright, J. (2014). Are we using blood pressure-lowering drugs appropriately? Perhaps now is the time for a change. *Journal of Human Hypertension*, **28**, 68–70.

Hagan, P. (2013). Eating walnuts twice a week could slash the risk of type 2 diabetes by a quarter. Associated Newspapers Ltd, London. Available at: http://www.dailymail.co.uk/health/article-2302326/Eating-walnuts-slash-type-2-diabetes-risk-research-suggests.html#ixzz3fOjvI46m (accessed 18 August 2015).

Hansard, Parliament Bill, HC Deb 11 November 1947 vol **444**, cc203–321. Available at: http://hansard.millbanksystems.com/commons/1947/nov/11/parliament-bill

Haw, S. and Gruer, L. (2007). Changes in exposure of adult non-smokers to secondhand smoke after implementation of smoke-free legislation in Scotland: national cross-sectional survey. *British Medical Journal*, **335**, 549.

Hawken, S.J., Greenwood, C.M., Hudson, T.J., et al. (2010). The utility and predictive value of combinations of low penetrance genes for screening and risk prediction of colorectal cancer. *Human Genetics*, **128**, 89–101.

Hennekens, C.H., Buring, J.E., and Mayrent, S.L. (1987). *Epidemiology in medicine*. Little, Brown Publishers, London.

Hertzman, C. and Frank, J. (2006). Biological pathways linking the social environment, developmental and health. In: Heymann, J., Hertzman, C., Barer, M.L., and Evans, R.G. (eds), *Healthier societies: from analysis to action*, pp. 35–57. Oxford University Press, Oxford.

Hertzman, C., Frank, J.W., and Evans, R.G. (1994). Heterogeneities in health status and the determinants of population health. In: Evans, R.G., Barer, M.L., and Marmor, T.R. (eds), *Why Are Some People Healthy and Others Not?*, pp. 67–92. Aldine-De Gruyter, Hawthorne, New York, NY.

Hertzman, C., Siddiqi, A.A., Hertzman, E., et al. (2010). Tackling inequality: get them while they're young. *British Medical Journal*, **340**, 346–8.

Hertzman, C. and Wiens, M. (1996). Child development and long-term outcomes: a population health perspective and summary of successful interventions. *Social Science and Medicine*, **43**, 1083–95.

Hill, A.B. (1965). The environment and disease: association or causation? *Proceedings of the Royal Society of Medicine*, **58**, 295–300.

Hill, S., Amos, A., Clifford, D., and Platt, S. (2014). Impact of tobacco control interventions on socioeconomic inequalities in smoking: review of the evidence. *Tobacco Control*, **23**, e89–97.

Hippisley-Cox, J. and Coupland, C. (2010). Individualising the risks of statins in men and women in England and Wales: population-based cohort study. *Heart*, **96**, 939–47.

Hope, J. (2012). Give statins to all over-50s: even the healthy should take heart drug, says British expert. Daily Mail, London. Available at: http://www.dailymail.co.uk/health/article-2194892/All-50s-statins-regardless-health-history-says-Oxford-professor.html#ixzz3fPBTUjif (accessed 18 August 2015).

Horowitz, H.S. (1996). The effectiveness of community water fluoridation in the United States. *Journal of Public Health Dentistry*, **56**, 253–8.

Huntingdon's Disease Society of America. (2016).What is Huntingdon's Disease? Available at:.http://www.hdsa.org/what-is-hd (Accessed 3 January2016).

Hutton, J.L. (2009). Number needed to treat and number needed to harm are not the best way to report and assess the results of randomised clinical trials. *British Journal of Haematology*, **146**, 27–30.

Independent UK Panel on Breast Cancer Screening (2012). The benefits and harms of breast cancer screening: an independent review. *Lancet*, **380**, 1778–86.

Ioannidis, J.P. (2005). Why most published research findings are false. *PLoS Medicine*, **2**, e124.

Janssens, A.C., Gwinn, M., Bradley, L.A., Oostra, B.A., van Duijn, C.M., and Khoury, M.J. (2008). A critical appraisal of the scientific basis of commercial genomic profiles used to assess health risks and personalize health interventions. *American Journal of Human Genetics*, **82**, 593–9.

Jepson, R.G., Williams, G., and Craig, J.C. (2012). Cranberries for preventing urinary tract infections. *Cochrane Database of Systematic Reviews*, Issue 10, Art. No.: CD001321.

Karha, J. and Topol, E.J. (2004). The sad story of Vioxx, and what we should learn from it. *Cleveland Clinical Journal of Medicine*, **71**, 933–4, 6, 8–9.

Katzman, R. (1993). Education and the prevalence of dementia and Alzheimer's disease. *Neurology*, **43**, 13–20.

Keating, D.P. and Hertzman, C. (1999). *Developmental health and the wealth of nations: social, biological, and educational dynamics*. Guilford Press, London.

Kohli, P. and Cannon, C.P. (2011). Statins and safety: can we finally be reassured? *Lancet*, **378**, 1980–1.

Krogsbøll, L.T., Jørgensen, K.J., Grønhøj Larsen, C., and Gøtzsche, P.C. (2012). General health checks in adults for reducing morbidity and mortality from disease. *Cochrane Database of Systematic Reviews*, Issue 10, Art.No.: CD009009.

Laguna, J. and **Carpenter, K.J.** (1951). Raw versus processed corn in niacin-deficient diets. *Journal of Nutrition*, **45**, 21–8.

Lang, T. and **Rayner, G.** (2007). Overcoming policy cacophony on obesity: an ecological public health framework for policymakers. *Obesity Reviews*, **8**(Suppl. 1), 165–81.

Laupacis, A., **Sackett, D.L.**, and **Roberts, R.S.** (1988). An assessment of clinically useful measures of the consequences of treatment. *New England Journal of Medicine*, **318**, 1728–33.

Ledingham, J.G.G. and Warrell, D.A. (eds.) (2000). *Concise Oxford textbook of medicine.* Oxford University Press, Oxford.

Little, J. and **Hawken, S.** (2010). On track? Using the Human Genome Epidemiology Roadmap. *Public Health Genomics*, **13**, 256–66.

Liu, S.F., **Shen, Q.**, **Dawsey, S.M.**, et al. (1994) Esophageal balloon cytology and subsequent risk of esophageal and gastric cancer. *International Journal of Cancer*, **57** (6):775-80.

Lloyd, S.M., **Stott, D.J.**, **de Craen, A.J.**, et al. (2013). Long-term effects of statin treatment in elderly people: extended follow-up of the PROspective Study of Pravastatin in the Elderly at Risk (PROSPER). *PLoS One*, **8**, e72642.

Lorenc, T., **Petticrew, M.**, **Welch, V.**, and **Tugwell, P.** (2013). What types of interventions generate inequalities? Evidence from systematic reviews. *Journal of Epidemiology Community Health*, **67**, 190–3.

Lynch, J.W., **Kaplan, G.A.**, and **Salonen, J.T.** (1997). Why do poor people behave poorly? Variation in adult health behaviours and psychosocial characteristics by stages of the socioeconomic lifecourse. *Social Science & Medicine*, **44**, 809–19.

Macedo, A.F., **Taylor, F.C.**, **Casas, J.P.**, **Adler, A.**, **Prieto-Merino, D.**, and **Ebrahim, S.** (2014). Unintended effects of statins from observational studies in the general population: systematic review and meta-analysis. *BMC Medicine*, **12**, 51.

Macintyre, S. (2007). Inequalities in health in Scotland: what are they and what can we do about them? MRC Social and Public Health Science Unit, Glasgow. Available at: http://www.sphsu.mrc.ac.uk/publications/occasional-papers.html (accessed 18 August 2015).

Mackenbach, J.P., **Kulhanova, I.**, **Menvielle, G.**, et al. (2015). Trends in inequalities in premature mortality: a study of 3.2 million deaths in 13 European countries. *Journal of Epidemiology Community Health*, **69**, 207–17; discussion 5–6.

Madlensky, L., **McLaughlin, J.R.**, **Carroll, J.C.**, **Goel, V.**, and **Frank, J.W.** (2005). Risks and benefits of population-based genetic testing for Mendelian subsets of common diseases were examined using the example of colorectal cancer risk. *Journal of Clinical Epidemiology*, **58**, 934–41.

Mandelblatt, J.S., **Cronin, K.A.**, **Bailey, S.**, et al. (2009). Effects of mammography screening under different screening schedules: model estimates of potential benefits and harms. *Annals of Internal Medicine*, **151**, 738–47.

Maningat, P., **Gordon, B.R.**, and **Breslow, J.L.** (2013). How do we improve patient compliance and adherence to long-term statin therapy? *Current Atherosclerosis Reports*, **15**, 291–9.

Marmot, M. (1997). Inequality, deprivation and alcohol use. *Addiction*, **92**, S13–20.

Marmot, M. (2010). *Fair society, healthy lives (the Marmot review)*. UCL Institute of Health Equity, London. Available at: http://www.instituteofhealthequity.org/projects/fair-society-healthy-lives-the-marmot-review (accessed 13 December 2015).

Marmot, M., Friel, S., Bell, R., Houweling, T.A., Taylor, S., and Commission on Social Determinants of Health (2008). Closing the gap in a generation: health equity through action on the social determinants of health. *Lancet*, **372**, 1661–9.

Martin, S.A., Boucher, M., Wright, J.M., and Saini, V. (2014). Mild hypertension in people at low risk. *British Medical Journal*, **349**, g5432.

McCombie, L., Lean, M.E., Haslam, D., and Counterweight Research Group (2012). Effective UK weight management services for adults. *Clinical Obesity*, **2**, 96–102.

McGill, R., Anwar, E., Orton, L., et al. (2015). Are interventions to promote healthy eating equally effective for all? Systematic review of socioeconomic inequalities in impact. *BMC Public Health*, **15**, 457–471.

McKeown, T. (1976). *The role of medicine: dream, mirage or nemesis?* Nuffield Provincial Hospitals Trust, London.

McLeod, K.S. (2000). Our sense of Snow: the myth of John Snow in medical geography. *Social Science Medicine*, **50**, 923–35.

McMaster University (2015). *Health Evidence*. McMaster University, Hamilton, Ontario. http://www.healthevidence.org/search-login.aspx (accessed 18 August 2015).

Miller, A.B. (2012). New data on prostate-cancer mortality after PSA screening. *New England Journal of Medicine*, **366**, 1047–8.

Miller, M.D., Marty, M.A., Broadwin, R., et al. (2007). The association between exposure to environmental tobacco smoke and breast cancer: a review by the California Environmental Protection Agency. *Preventive Medicine*, **44**, 93–106.

Mills, E.J., Wu, P., Chong, G., et al. (2011). Efficacy and safety of statin treatment for cardiovascular disease: a network meta-analysis of 170,255 patients from 76 randomized trials. *Quarterly Journal of Medicine*, **104**, 109–24.

Moodie, M., Sheppard, L., Sacks, G., Keating, C., and Flego, A. (2013). Cost-effectiveness of fiscal policies to prevent obesity. *Current Obesity Reports*, **2**, 211–24.

Mooney, J.D., Jepson, R., Frank, J., and Geddes, R. (2015). Obesity prevention in Scotland: a policy analysis using the ANGELO framework. *Obesity Facts*, **8**, 273–81.

Morabia, A. (2007). Epidemiological methods and concepts in the nineteenth century and their influences on the twentieth century. In: Holland, W.W., Olsen, J., and Florey, C.d.V. (eds), *The development of modern epidemiology: personal reports from those who were there*, pp. 17–29. Oxford University Press, Oxford.

Mostafa, T. and Green, A. (2012). Measuring the impact of universal pre-school education and care on literacy performance scores. Centre for Learning and Life Chances in Knowledge Economies and Societies, London. Available at: http://www.llakes.org/wp-content/uploads/2012/07/36.-Mostafa-Green.pdf (accessed 18 August 2015).

Moyer, V.A. and U. S. Preventive Services Task Force (2012). Screening for prostate cancer: U.S. Preventive Services Task Force recommendation statement. *Annals of Internal Medicine*, **157**, 120–34.

Mozaffarian, D. and Clarke, R. (2009). Quantitative effects on cardiovascular risk factors and coronary heart disease risk of replacing partially hydrogenated vegetable oils with other fats and oils. *European Journal of Clinical Nutrition*, **63**, S22–33.

Mozaffarian, D., Lemaitre, R.N., King, I.B., et al. (2013). Plasma phospholipid long-chain omega-3 fatty acids and total and cause-specific mortality in older adults: a cohort study. *Annals of Internal Medicine*, **158**, 515–25.

Mozaffarian, D. and Ludwig, D.S. (2015). The 2015 US dietary guidelines: lifting the ban on total dietary fat. *Journal of the American Medical Association*, **313**, 2421–2.

National Comprehensive Cancer Network (2014). Prostate cancer early detection. version 1.2014. National Comprehensive Cancer Network, Fort Washington, PA. Available at: http://www.tri-kobe.org/nccn/guideline/urological/english/prostate_detection.pdf (accessed 18 August 2015).

National Institute for Health and Care Excellence (2006a). Brief interventions and referral for smoking cessation. National Institute for Health and Care Excellence, Manchester. Available at: http://www.nice.org.uk/guidance/ph1 (accessed 18 August 2015).

National Institute for Health and Care Excellence, 2010. Alcohol-use disorders: preventing harmful drinking. National Institute for Health and Care Excellence, Manchester. Available at: http://www.nice.org.uk/guidance/ph24 (accessed 18 August 2015).

National Institute for Health and Care Excellence (2014). Lipid modification: cardiovascular risk assessment and the modification of blood lipids for the primary and secondary prevention of cardiovascular disease. National Institute for Health and Care Excellence, London. Available at: https://www.nice.org.uk/guidance/cg181 (accessed 18 August 2015).

National Institute for Health and Clinical Excellence (2006b). Obesity: guidance on the prevention of overweight and obesity in adults and children. National Institute for Health and Clinical Excellence, London. Available at: http://www.nice.org.uk/guidance/cg43 (accessed 18 August 2015).

Nelson, H.D., Tyne, K., Naik, A., et al. (2009). Screening for breast cancer: an update for the U.S. Preventive Services Task Force. *Annals of Internal Medicine*, **151**, 727–37, W237–42.

NHS Choices (2012). Cranberry juice 'won't prevent' bladder infections. GOV. UK, London. Available at: http://www.nhs.uk/news/2012/10October/Pages/Cranberry-juice-no-good-in-preventing-bladder-infections.aspx (accessed 18 August 2015).

NHS Screening Programmes (2015). Antenatal and newborn screening: introduction. Public Health England, London. Available at: http://cpd.screening.nhs.uk/cms.php?folder=3136 (accessed 18 August 2015).

Nores, M. and **Barnett, W.S.** (2010). Benefits of early childhood interventions across the world: (under) investing in the very young. *Economics of Education Review*, **29**, 271–82.

Nussbaum, R.L., **McInnes, R.R.**, and **Willard, H.F.** (2001). *Thompson & Thompson Genetics in medicine*, 6th edn. W.B. Saunders, Philadelphia, PA.

Office for National Statistics (2013). One third of babies born in 2013 are expected to live to 100. Office for National Statistics, Newport. Available at: http://www.ons.gov.uk/ons/rel/lifetables/historic-and-projected-data-from-the-period-and-cohort-lifetables/2012-based/sty-babies-living-to-100.html (accessed 18 August 2015).

Ogden, L.G., **He, J.**, **Lydick, E.**, and **Whelton, P.K.** (2000). Long-term absolute benefit of lowering blood pressure in hypertensive patients according to the JNC VI risk stratification. *Hypertension*, **35**, 539–43.

Ogilvie, D., **Fayter, D.**, **Petticrew, M.**, et al. (2008). The harvest plot: a method for synthesising evidence about the differential effects of interventions. *BMC Medical Research Methodology*, **8**, 8.

Omenn, G.S., **Goodman, G.E.**, **Thornquist, M.D.**, et al. (1996). Risk factors for lung cancer and for intervention effects in CARET, the beta-carotene and retinol efficacy trial. *Journal of the National Cancer Institute*, **88**, 1550–9.

Ostry, A.S. and **Frank, J.** (2010). Was Thomas McKeown right for the wrong reasons? *Critical Public Health*, **20**, 233–43.

Oxford English Dictionary (2015). 'hygiene, n.'. Oxford University Press, Oxford.

Pan, A., **Sun, Q.**, **Manson, J.E.**, **Willett, W.C.**, and **Hu, F.B.** (2013). Walnut consumption is associated with lower risk of type 2 diabetes in women. *Journal of Nutrition*, **143**, 512–18.

Parliamentary Office of Science and Technology (2012). Consumer genetic testing. Houses of Parliament, London. Available at: www.parliament.uk/briefing-papers/POST-PN-407.pdf (accessed 18 August 2015).

Patton, M.Q. (1990). *Qualitative research & evaluation methods*, 2nd edn. Sage Publications, Inc., Thousand Oaks, CA.

Pawson, R. (2013). *The science of evaluation: a realist manifesto*. Sage Publications, London.

Pawson, R. & **Tilley, N.** (1997). *Realistic evaluation*. Sage Publications, London.

Pell, J.P., **Haw, S.**, **Cobbe, S.**, et al. (2008). Smoke-free legislation and hospitalizations for acute coronary syndrome. *New England Journal of Medicine*, **359**, 482–91.

Peto, R., **Doll, R.**, **Buckley, J.D.**, and **Sporn, M.B.** (1981). Can dietary beta-carotene materially reduce human cancer rates? *Nature*, **290**, 201–8.

Petrosino, A., **Turpin-Petrosino, C.**, **Hollis-Peel Meghan, E.**, and **Lavenberg Julia, G.** (2013). 'Scared straight' and other juvenile awareness programs for preventing juvenile delinquency. *Campbell Systematic Reviews*, Volume **9**, Issue 5.

Pollan, M. (2008). *In defense of food: an eater's manifesto*. Penguin Press, New York.

Porta, M.S. (2008). *A dictionary of epidemiology*, 6th edn. Oxford University Press, New York.

Public Health England (2015). *The eatwell plate*. NHS Choices, London.

Raffle, A.E. and **Gray, J.A.M.** (2007). *Screening: evidence and practice*. Oxford University Press, Oxford.

Reddy, K.S. and **Yusuf, S.** (1998). Emerging epidemic of cardiovascular disease in developing countries. *Circulation*, **97**, 596–601.

Reiner, Z. (2013). Statins in the primary prevention of cardiovascular disease. *Nature Review: Cardiology*, **10**, 453–64.

Reitz, C., Brayne, C., and **Mayeux, R.** (2011). Epidemiology of Alzheimer disease. *Nature Review: Neurology*, **7**, 137–52.

Ridker, P.M., Pradhan, A., MacFadyen, J.G., Libby, P., and **Glynn, R.J.** (2012). Cardiovascular benefits and diabetes risks of statin therapy in primary prevention: an analysis from the JUPITER trial. *Lancet*, **380**, 565–71.

Riley, K.P., Snowdon, D.A., Desrosiers, M.F., and **Markesbery, W.R.** (2005). Early life linguistic ability, late life cognitive function, and neuropathology: findings from the Nun Study. *Neurobiology of Aging*, **26**, 341–7.

Riley, L.W., Raphael, E., and **Faerstein, E.** (2013). Obesity in the United States—dysbiosis from exposure to low-dose antibiotics? *Frontiers in Public Health*, **1**, 69.

Roberts, M. (2012). Cranberry juice 'can protect against urine infections'. British Broadcasting Corporation News, London. Available at: http://www.bbc.co.uk/news/health-18768320 (accessed 18 August 2015).

Roberts, N.J., Vogelstein, J.T., Parmigiani, G., Kinzler, K.W., Vogelstein, B., and **Velculescu, V.E.** (2012). The predictive capacity of personal genome sequencing. *Science Translational Medicine*, **4**, 133ra58.

Roddam, A.W., Pirie, K., Pike, M.C., et al. (2007). Active and passive smoking and the risk of breast cancer in women aged 36-45 years: a population based case-control study in the UK. *British Journal of Cancer*, **97**, 434–9.

Rogers, E.M. (2002). Diffusion of preventive innovations. *Addictive Behaviors*, **27**, 989–93.

Rose, G. (1985). Sick individuals and sick populations. *International Journal of Epidemiology*, **14**, 32–8.

Rose, G. (2008). *The strategy of preventive medicine*. Oxford University Press, Oxford.

Roseman, M., Turner, E.H., Lexchin, J., Coyne, J.C., Bero, L.A., and **Thombs, B.D.** (2012). Reporting of conflicts of interest from drug trials in Cochrane reviews: cross sectional study. *British Medical Journal*, **345**, e5155.

Rossouw, J.E., Anderson, G.L., Prentice, R.L., et al. (2002). Risks and benefits of estrogen plus progestin in healthy postmenopausal women: principal results From the Women's Health Initiative randomized controlled trial. *Journal of the American Medical Association*, **288**, 321–33.

Rothman, K.J., Greenland, S., and **Lash, T.L.** (2008). *Modern epidemiology*, 3rd edn. Lippincott Williams & Wilkins, Philadelphia, PA.

Sacks, O.W. (1997). *The island of the colorblind*. A.A. Knopf, New York, NY.

Sanson-Fisher, R.W., D'Este, C.A., Carey, M.L., Noble, N., and **Paul, C.L.** (2014). Evaluation of systems-oriented public health interventions: alternative research designs. *Annual Review of Public Health,* **35,** 9–27.

Sartorius, N., Jablensky, A., Korten, A., et al. (1986). Early manifestations and first-contact incidence of schizophrenia in different cultures. A preliminary report on the initial evaluation phase of the WHO Collaborative Study on determinants of outcome of severe mental disorders. *Psychological Medicine,* **16,** 909–28.

Sattar, N., Preiss, D., Murray, H.M., et al. (2010). Statins and risk of incident diabetes: a collaborative meta-analysis of randomised statin trials. *Lancet,* **375,** 735–42.

Schröder, F.H., Hugosson, J., Roobol, M.J., et al. (2009). Screening and prostate-cancer mortality in a randomized European study. *New England Journal of Medicine,* **360,** 1320–8.

Schröder, F.H., Hugosson, J., Roobol, M.J., et al. (2012). Prostate-cancer mortality at 11 years of follow-up. *New England Journal of Medicine,* **366,** 981–90.

Schulz, M.D., Atay, C., Heringer, J., et al. (2014). High-fat-diet-mediated dysbiosis promotes intestinal carcinogenesis independently of obesity. *Nature,* **514,** 508–12.

Schwartz, J.L. (2012). The first rotavirus vaccine and the politics of acceptable risk. *Milbank Quarterly,* **90,** 278–310.

Scottish Government (2014). Long term monitoring of health inequalities: headline indicators—October 2014. Scottish Government, Edinburgh. Available at: http://www.gov.scot/Publications/2014/10/7902/7 (accessed 18 August 2015).

Semple, S., Creely, K.S., Maji, A., Miller, B.G., and **Ayres, J.G.** (2007). Secondhand smoke levels in Scottish pubs: the effect of smoke-free legislation. *Tobacco Control,* **16,** 127–32.

Sijbrands, E.J., Westendorp, R.G., Defesche, J.C., de Meier, P.H., Smelt, A.H., and **Kastelein, J.J.** (2001). Mortality over two centuries in large pedigree with familial hypercholesterolaemia: family tree mortality study. *British Medical Journal,* **322,** 1019–23.

Skinner, A.C. and **Skelton, J.A.** (2014). Prevalence and trends in obesity and severe obesity among children in the United States, 1999–2012. *Journal of the American Medical Association of Pediatrics,* **168,** 561–6.

Smeeth, L., Haines, A., and **Ebrahim, S.** (1999). Numbers needed to treat derived from meta-analyses—sometimes informative, usually misleading. *British Medical Journal,* **318,** 1548–51.

Smith, R. (2006). Conflicts of interest: how money clouds objectivity. *Journal of the Royal Society of Medicine,* **99,** 292–7.

Social Science Research Unit (2009). Welcome to the EPPI-Centre. Institute of Education, London. Available at: https://eppi.ioe.ac.uk/cms/ (accessed 18 August 2015).

Spencer, P.S., Ludolph, A.C., and **Kisby, G.E.** (1993). Neurologic diseases associated with use of plant components with toxic potential. *Environmental Research,* **62,** 106–13.

Stone, N.J., Robinson, J.G., Lichtenstein, A.H., et al. (2014). 2013 ACC/AHA guideline on the treatment of blood cholesterol to reduce atherosclerotic cardiovascular risk in adults: a report of the American College of Cardiology/American Heart Association Task Force on Practice Guidelines. *Circulation*, **129**, S1–45.

Stuckler, D., McKee, M., Ebrahim, S., and Basu, S. (2012). Manufacturing epidemics: the role of global producers in increased consumption of unhealthy commodities including processed foods, alcohol, and tobacco. *PLoS Medicine*, **9**, e1001235.

Swerdlow, D.I., Preiss, D., Kuchenbaecker, K.B., et al. (2015). HMG-coenzyme A reductase inhibition, type 2 diabetes, and bodyweight: evidence from genetic analysis and randomised trials. *Lancet*, **385**, 351–61.

Tate, J.E., Burton, A.H., Boschi-Pinto, C., et al. (2012). 2008 estimate of worldwide rotavirus-associated mortality in children younger than 5 years before the introduction of universal rotavirus vaccination programmes: a systematic review and meta-analysis. *Lancet: Infectious Diseases*, **12**, 136–41.

Telegraph (2013). Walnuts cuts diabetes risk by one quarter. Telegraph Media Group, London. Available at: http://www.telegraph.co.uk/news/health/news/9964942/ Walnuts-cuts-diabetes-risk-by-one-quarter.html (accessed 18 August 2015).

Temple, J.A. and Reynolds, A.J. (2007). Benefits and costs of investments in preschool education: Evidence from the Child–Parent Centers and related programs. *Economics of Education Review*, **26**, 126–44.

Thompson, R., Gerada, C., Haslam, D., et al. (2014). Concerns about the latest NICE draft guidance on statins [letter sent 10th June 2014]. National Institute for Health and Care Excellence, London. Available at: http://www.nice.org.uk/Media/Default/ News/NICE-statin-letter.pdf (accessed 18 August 2015).

Todd, J., Fishaut, M., Kapral, F., and Welch, T. (1978). Toxic-shock syndrome associated with phage-group-I staphylococci. *Lancet*, **2**, 1116–18.

Toronto Working Group on Cholesterol Policy, Naylor, C.D., Basinski, A., Frank, J.W., and Rachlis, M.M. (1990). Asymptomatic hypercholesterolemia: a clinical policy review *Journal of Clinical Epidemiology*, **43**, 1021–121.

Tugwell, P., de Savigny, D., Hawker, G., and Robinson, V. (2006). Applying clinical epidemiological methods to health equity: the equity effectiveness loop. *British Medical Journal*, **332**, 358–61.

Tugwell, P., Petticrew, M., Kristjansson, E., et al. (2010). Assessing equity in systematic reviews: realising the recommendations of the Commission on Social Determinants of Health. *British Medical Journal*, **341**, c4739.

UCL Institute of Health Equity (2014). Review of social determinants and the health divide in the WHO European Region: final report. World Health Organization Regional Office for Europe, Copenhagen. Available at: http://www.euro.who.int/ __data/assets/pdf_file/0004/251878/Review-of-social-determinants-and-the-health-divide-in-the-WHO-European-Region-FINAL-REPORT.pdf (accessed 18 August 2015).

US Department of Agriculture, US Department of Health and Human Service (2015). Scientific report of the 2015 dietary guidelines advisory committee. U.S.

Department of Agriculture and U.S. Department of Health and Human Service, Washington, D.C. Available at: http://www.health.gov/dietaryguidelines/2015-scientific-report/pdfs/scientific-report-of-the-2015-dietary-guidelines-advisory-committee.pdf (accessed 18 August 2015).

US Federal Trade Commission (2014). Direct-to-consumer genetic tests. Federal Trade Commission, Washington, DC. Available at: http://www.consumer.ftc. gov/articles/0166-direct-consumer-genetic-tests (accessed 18 August 2015).

US Food and Drug Administration (2015a). FDA cuts trans fat in processed foods. U.S. Food and Drug Administration, Silver Spring, MD. Available at: http:// www.fda.gov/downloads/ForConsumers/ConsumerUpdates/UCM451467.pdf (accessed 18 August 2015).

US Food and Drug Administration (2015b). Final determination regarding partially hydrogenated oils. *Federal Register*, **80**, 34650–70.

US Preventive Services Task Force (2002). Postmenopausal hormone replacement therapy for primary prevention of chronic conditions: recommendations and rationale. *Annals of Internal Medicine*, **137**, 834–9.

US Preventive Services Task Force (2007). Final recommendation statement: lipid disorders in children: screening. U.S. Preventive Services Task Force, Rockville, MD. Available at: http://www.uspreventiveservicestaskforce.org/Page/Document/ RecommendationStatementFinal/lipid-disorders-in-children-screening (accessed 18 August 2015).

US Preventive Services Task Force (2008). Final recommendation statement: colorectal cancer: screening. U.S. Preventive Services Task Force, Rockville, MD. Available at: http://www.uspreventiveservicestaskforce.org/Page/Document/ RecommendationStatementFinal/colorectal-cancer-screening (accessed 18 August 2015).

US Preventive Services Task Force (2009a). Final recommendation statement: tobacco use in adults and pregnant women: counseling and interventions. U.S. Preventive Services Task Force, Rockville, MD. Available at: http://www.uspreventiveservicestaskforce.org/Page/Document/ RecommendationStatementFinal/tobacco-use-in-adults-and-pregnant-women-counseling-and-interventions (accessed 18 August 2015).

US Preventive Services Task Force (2009b). Screening for breast cancer: US Preventive Services Task Force recommendation statement. *Annals of Internal Medicine*, **151**, 716–26, W-236.

US Preventive Services Task Force (2012a). Final recommendation statement: cervical cancer. U.S. Preventive Services Task Force, Rockville, MD. Available at: http://www.uspreventiveservicestaskforce.org/Page/Document/ RecommendationStatementFinal/cervical-cancer-screening (accessed 18 August 2015).

US Preventive Services Task Force (2012b). Final recommendation statement: prostate cancer: screening. U.S. Preventive Services Task Force, Rockville, MD. Available at: http://www.uspreventiveservicestaskforce.org/Page/Document/

RecommendationStatementFinal/prostate-cancer-screening (accessed 18 August 2015).

US **Preventive Services Task Force** (2013a). Final recommendation statement: alcohol misuse: screening and behavioral counseling interventions in primary care. U.S. Preventive Services Task Force, Rockville, MD. Available at: http://www.uspreventiveservicestaskforce.org/Page/Document/RecommendationStatementFinal/alcohol-misuse-screening-and-behavioral-counseling-interventions-in-primary-care (accessed 18 August 2015).

US **Preventive Services Task Force** (2013b). Final recommendation statement: lung cancer. U. S. Preventive Services Task Force, Rockville, MD. Available at: http://www.uspreventiveservicestaskforce.org/Page/Document/RecommendationStatementFinal/lung-cancer-screening (accessed 18 August 2015).

US **Preventive Services Task Force**, 2015. Home. USPSTF Program Office, Rockville, MD. Available at: http://www.uspreventiveservicestaskforce.org/ (accessed 18 August 2015).

Vahouny, G.V., Connor, W.E., Roy, T., Lin, D.S., and **Gallo, L.L.** (1981). Lymphatic absorption of shellfish sterols and their effects on cholesterol absorption. *American Journal of Clinical Nutrition*, **34**, 507–13.

Valls-Pedret, C., Sala-Vila, A., Serra-Mir, M., et al. (2015). Mediterranean diet and age-related cognitive decline: A randomized clinical trial. *Journal of the American Medical Association Internal Medicine*, **175**, 1094–103.

Vineis, P., Schulte, P., and **McMichael, A.J.** (2001). Misconceptions about the use of genetic tests in populations. *Lancet*, **357**, 709–12.

Vinten-Johansen, P., Brody, H., Paneth, N., Rachman, S., and **Rip, M.** (2003). *Cholera, chloroform, and the science of medicine: a life of John Snow*. Oxford University Press, Oxford.

von Mutius, E. (2007). Allergies, infections and the hygiene hypothesis—the epidemiological evidence. *Immunobiology*, **212**, 433–9.

Wald, N. and **Morris, J.** (2014). Refining the American guidelines for prevention of cardiovascular disease. *Lancet*, **383**, 598.

Wald, N.J., Simmonds, M., and **Morris, J.K.** (2011). Screening for future cardiovascular disease using age alone compared with multiple risk factors and age. *PLoS One*, **6**, e18742.

Wang, C-H., Fang, C-C., Chen, N-C., et al. (2012). Cranberry-containing products for prevention of urinary tract infections in susceptible populations: A systematic review and meta-analysis of randomized controlled trials. *Archives of Internal Medicine*, **172**, 988–96.

Wang, Y.F., Beydoun, M.A., Liang, L., Caballero, B., and **Kumanyika, S.K.** (2008). Will all Americans become overweight or obese? Estimating the progression and cost of the US obesity epidemic. *Obesity*, **16**, 2323–30.

Welch, H.G., Schwartz, L., and **Woloshin, S.** (2011). *Overdiagnosed: making people sick in the pursuit of health*. Beacon Press, Boston, MA.

Welch, V., Petticrew, M., Tugwell, P., et al. (2012). PRISMA-Equity 2012 extension: reporting guidelines for systematic reviews with a focus on health equity. *PLoS Medicine*, **9**, e1001333.

Westlake, S.J. and Frank, J.W. (1987). Testicular self-examination: an argument against routine teaching. *Family Practice*, **4**, 143–8.

Whitehead, M. (2000). William Farr's legacy to the study of inequalities in health. *Bulletin World Health Organization*, **78**, 86–7.

Wilkinson, R. and Marmot, M. (2003). *Social determinants of health: the solid facts*, 2nd edn. World Health Organization, Regional Office for Europe, Copenhagen.

Willms, J.D. (2003). Literacy proficiency of youth: evidence of converging socioeconomic gradients. *International Journal of Educational Research*, **39**, 247–52.

Wilson, J.M.G. and Jungner, G. (1968). *Principles and practice of screening for disease*. World Health Organization, Geneva.

World Cancer Research Fund/American Institute for Cancer Research (2007). *Food, nutrition, physical activity, and the prevention of cancer: a global perspective*. AICR, Washington DC. Available at: http://www.dietandcancerreport.org/cancer_resource_center/downloads/Second_Expert_Report_full.pdf (accessed 18 August 2015).

World Health Organization (2008). Closing the gap in a generation. World Health Organization. Available at: http://apps.who.int/bookorders/anglais/detart1.jsp?codlan=1&codcol=15&codcch=741 (accessed 18 August 2015).

Wright, J.M. and Musini, V.M. (2009). First-line drugs for hypertension. *Cochrane Database of Systematic Reviews*, Issue 3. Art.No.: CD001841.

Wynder, E.L. and Graham, E.A. (1950). Tobacco smoking as a possible etiologic factor in bronchiogenic carcinoma; a study of 684 proved cases. *Journal of the American Medical Association*, **143**, 329–36.

Young, T.K. (1998). *Population health: concepts and methods*. Oxford University Press, New York.

Index